# Patient Participation in Program Planning: A Manual for Therapists

# Patient Participation in Program Planning: A Manual for Therapists

**OTTO D. PAYTON, Ph.D., P.T.**
Professor of Physical Therapy
School of Allied Health Professions
Medical College of Virginia
Virginia Commonwealth University
Richmond, Virginia

**MARK N. OZER, M.D.**
Assistant Chief, Spinal Cord Injury Service
Hunter Holmes McGuire VA Medical Center
Associate Professor of Neurology
Medical College of Virginia
Virginia Commonwealth University
Richmond, Virginia

**CRAIG E. NELSON, M.S., O.T.R.**
Associate Professor of Occupational Therapy
School of Allied Health Professions
Medical College of Virginia
Virginia Commonwealth University
Richmond, Virginia

 **F. A. Davis Company • Philadelphia**

Copyright © 1990 by F. A. Davis Company

Printed in the United States of America

Last digit indicates print number: 10 9 8 7 6 5 4 3 2 1

**Library of Congress Cataloging-in-Publication Data**

Payton, Otto D.
Patient participation in planning  :  a manual for therapists  /
  Otto Payton, Craig Nelson, Mark N. Ozer.
    p.    cm.
Includes bibliographies and index.
ISBN 0-8036-6803-1
1. Physical therapy—Planning—Handbooks, manuals, etc.
2. Occupational therapy—Planning—Handbooks, manuals, etc.
3. Patient compliance—Handbooks, manuals, etc.    I. Nelson,
Craig.    II. Ozer, Mark N.    III. Title
[DNLM:    1. Patient    Participation.    2. Rehabilitation—
methods.    WB 320 P347p]
RM701.P39    1989
615.8'2—dc20
DNLM/DLC
for Library of Congress                                                89-16154
                                                                              CIP

To Cindy and Brent
C.N.

and

To Martha
M.N.O.

# Contents

# Introduction

This book is designed for use by students in physical and occupational therapy or by therapists in the context of an in-service training program, including those who wish to pursue such training by self-study. The final goal of this educational program is to be able to demonstrate the knowledge and skills needed to involve patients/clients in a fruitful and productive way in the management of their own therapeutic program.

The method for involving patients in planning arose out of my experience with a large variety of persons with disabilities. The adaptation of those methods to physical and occupational therapy and the development of methods for educating professionals in those fields came about in conjunction with my colleagues in writing this book as we worked with students over several years.

The assumptions that underlie this method for patient participation in planning have been based upon the experience that goals that arise from the persons involved are more likely to receive the investment of energy that will bring them to achievement. It is the patient alone who can ultimately determine whether a goal is worth working for; and, as much as is consistent with clarity, the goals should be stated in the patient's own language. Once the goals are so stated, the patient can in turn participate in the ongoing process of evaluation of outcomes and of the activities used to achieve those outcomes. Patient participation in planning can thus underlie the entire therapeutic process, making it more effective and more efficient.

In an important sense, the process being described is based also on recognition of the values of self-determination and the worth of the individual. The goal is to integrate the therapist's competence in interpreting signs and symptoms and in the technical application of treatments, while emphasizing that planning and evaluative skills must be shared with the client. It is the client who must ultimately be prepared to deal with his or her problems and to do so not only in the short term but, in many instances, throughout the rest of his or her life. Patient participation in planning can be the context for learning an important skill for his or her future, along with the more traditional skills such as activities of daily living and mobility.

There are several stages recommended for learning to use the planning system described in this book. The first step is, perhaps, the most unique. It requires exercises and other methods by which the person using the book learns first to apply the method and see results in his or her own life. The context for application to oneself is the reader's planning in relation to learning to master this particular approach for working with patients/clients. This procedure accomplishes two things: First, it makes the book real and useful to the reader's professional role by providing a tool for personal planning. Second, it enables the reader to experience the process which he or she will later help the patient to learn for himself or herself. Experiencing a modality first on oneself is a frequently used educational technique in therapy education; it is very relevant here. Throughout this book the terms "book" and "course" will be considered to be synonymous.

Having experienced the planning process personally, the reader is then led to experiment with the process in interviews with others. Finally, the reader will use the process with clients in a therapeutic setting to involve the people with disabilities in defining their own concerns, goals, and plans for rehabilitating their own lives. *Patient* and/or *client* are used interchangeably for the person involved in the therapeutic program so as to reflect differences in terminology in various professional settings. In light of the different settings in which this course has been used, the reader is referred to at times as a student, therapist, or clinician.

As one grows in the use of this approach, the number of questions one addresses becomes greater. The skills sought, therefore, are to be able to define one's own answers to a series of planning questions, then to enable patients to do the same. This is done in stages which can be reflected in components of a course that will extend over time and be integrated with concomitant increase in a student's clinical skills and experience.

In the first stage, the planning questions are:

1. What concerns you at this time? (problems)
2. What would you like to see happen? (goals)

Having now elicited patient input toward the definition of a goal, at a subsequent stage the goals are evaluated through an additional question:

3. What had been accomplished in relation to the goals? (outcomes)

Now the first two questions as to concerns and goals can be restated as well as the time line for reevaluation, but in light of the changes that may have occurred since they were first addressed.

At a still later stage for the training of both the student/therapist and with any one patient, in addition to the question as to outcomes, one may ask the question as to the means by which those outcomes were achieved:

4. What may have helped to bring about those results? (methods)

Although therapists are accustomed to asking this question, it is unusual to do so with the patient to the extent that the person with the disabilities could thus become a participant in the design of the therapeutic program. Once again, concerns and goals may be reviewed at this stage. The therapist and the patient now have data from the patient with which to construct an entire collaborative *plan*, based upon the experience of the methods that have been helpful.

5. What is the plan?

This fifth question will incorporate goals, means, and time line. Patient participation in all these aspects completes the development of skills in the planning process.

The procedure for answering each of these questions involves three basic steps: to *explore* and identify at least three alternatives; to make a *selection* on some basis such as priority; and then to *specify* the selection. The criteria for each of these steps of exploration, selection, and specification can be defined differently in answer to any one of these questions; and one may evaluate the degree to which each of these steps is performed. See Figure I–1 for an overall description of the entire process whereby the patient becomes successively involved in the entire set of questions.

At each stage of development in the use of these planning questions, the professional can share the skill acquired in planning for self by enabling another person such as a patient/client to answer these same questions. To help that other person answer the questions, a new degree of awareness is neces-

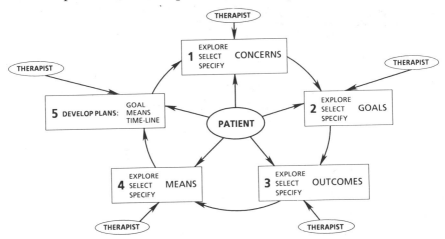

**FIGURE I–1.** Patient participation in program planning.

xi

sary in addition to the skill of answering the questions for oneself. The professional must be aware of the degree to which the answers arise from the patient rather than the professional. Ideally, one strives for "maximal" involvement on the part of the client consistent with the other objectives of adequate exploration, selection, and specification. If the therapeutic relationship is short term, one may merely seek client participation in several of the questions. A longer-term relationship may seek to expand client participation in answering the entire set of questions or even to the extent of the client asking the questions of oneself independent of any professional.

This book arose out of my work with a series of courses for students in physical and occupational therapy at undergraduate, graduate, and in-service levels. As the courses developed, they involved many students over several years. Each group of students provided new insights and made contributions to the focus of our work. One instance is that all the examples used in this book are real-life situations experienced by students or clinicians. It is to those students too numerous to mention by name that we dedicate this book. The hope is that they will use the ideas exemplified in this book to continue to grow in their professional lives by helping their clients grow in their own skills.

Mark N. Ozer, M.D.

# Section
# *one*

The chapters in this first section of the book are designed to follow the sequence of a course. Each chapter in turn follows the pattern of the planning process: The goals of that chapter are discussed and then the issues (or concerns) that may relate to those goals. Each chapter ends with a set of exercises and examples. The first of each set applies the content of that chapter to oneself as a student with examples of how others have used that very exercise. Readers are encouraged to copy the forms used and then to practice the skills discussed in each chapter. Finally, each chapter contains suggestions and examples of application of the content of that chapter to patients.

Chapter 1 provides the overall background and rationale for the course. The exercise at the end provides the student/therapist with the first opportunity to participate in the design of a course as a model for later use of these same questions with patient/client in the design of a therapeutic program. The exercise at the end of Chapter 1 explores the question of concerns. Chapter 2 prepares the reader to specify the goals for one's educational program as a prerequisite for doing so with patients. Chapter 3 deals with the evaluation of outcome by the student and then with a patient as part of an ongoing cycle of planning/evaluation and revision. Similarly, Chapter 4 deals with the question as to methods by which those outcomes were achieved and the use of that information as part of a total *plan*. Now that all 5 questions have been introduced, Chapter 4 also illustrates how one may choose to use one or another of the questions in day-to-day work with patients without necessarily using the entire sequence.

While the first 4 chapters present the knowledge and skills needed to involve patients in a meaningful way in their own therapeutic program planning, we believe it necessary, particularly for the entry-level student, to go beyond merely reading and to practice applying this process to oneself, peers,

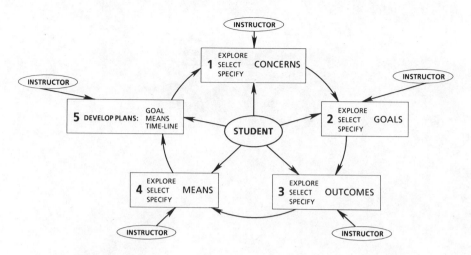

**FIGURE 1.** Student participation in educational planning.

and patients. Such practice is optimally integrated with clinical education. Concepts unclear at first will become more relevant with increasing clinical experience. Those who are already at work in clinical settings can put their learning into practice with more immediate results. Since clinics and clinical supervisors vary in their approach to problem solving with patients, the process described in this book can be modified for use in any clinical setting. Figure 1 illustrates the relationship between the instructor and the student/therapist as analogous to that of the therapist and the patient described earlier in Figure I-1.

# 1

# *The Educational Plan*

## WHAT IS THE OVERALL PROBLEM?

The issue of patient "compliance" to instructions given by health professionals is a serious problem. DiMatteo and DiNicola,[1] for example, have provided a detailed summary and discussion of the literature on patient compliance with prescribed treatment regimens. The news is not good. Patients follow a physician's instructions less than 50% of the time if treatment is aimed at long-term prevention. The percentage following instructions is considerably higher (in the range of 75%) if treatment is directed to relieve signs and symptoms that are of concern to the patient. Although most studies have dealt with the use of medication, there are some that have examined patient follow-through with exercise programs and other health behavior recommendations of health practitioners other than physicians.[2] Dishman and colleagues[3] have estimated, for example, that 50% of those who start general exercise programs discontinue them within 6 months. On the other hand, knowing that there would be a re-evaluation increased long-term follow-through (12 weeks) to an exercise program.[4]

Similar studies have dealt with the usage of equipment prescribed by occupational therapists. In a follow-up study, Allen[5] found that 43% of persons with quadriplegia continued to use their wrist-driven flexor hinge splint. Others[6] have found that 60% of persons with rheumatoid arthritis carried out a prescribed splint program. Considerably more successful was the use of adaptive equipment by persons undergoing hip arthroplasty. The largest percentage of persons used their equipment "always." The success was attributed

3

to the use of a thorough assessment procedure, but it may be noted that the therapist and the patient jointly set postdischarge goals.[7]

The importance of confronting this problem is its effect on the outcomes of health care. Failure to follow through with plans may jeopardize the person's health. It affects the quality and outcomes of health care and increases the costs of health care by decreasing its effectiveness. It also interferes with research intended to determine the efficacy of treatments.

Part of the problem may be attributed to the incongruence between the goals stated by patients and those of their therapists in a rehabilitation unit.[9] The patients tended to have such functional goals as "walking," whereas the therapist's goals were in physiologic terms such as "increased strength in the quadriceps muscle." When one compared treatment goals set by occupational therapists with those indicated by patients, there was frequent lack of agreement as to treatment goals of persons with quadriplegia.[10]

Incongruence often results when the therapist concentrates on the anatomic/physiologic/kinesiologic level of *impairment* while the patient focuses on the *disability* resulting from such an impairment.[11,12] For example, the same objective impairment resulting from an injury to the hand produces far different disabilities in a radio announcer than in a pianist. One should consider not only the degree of objective impairment but the interaction of that impairment with the person, his or her history and goals, and the environment in which that person seeks to function.[13]

Given this lack of congruence, many patients may not see the relevance of the therapeutic program to their goals, and so participation is compromised. Measurement of the degree of accomplishment of the goals by patients is also more likely if the goals are stated in terms within the patient's set of experience. Such participation by patients in the process of assessment of the accomplishment of goals helps the patient continue to put out the effort necessary for continued success; it helps patients cope.[11,14]

DiMatteo and DiNicola[1] state that follow-through is improved when patients' expectations regarding their treatment are met, which is more likely to occur when there is agreement between the expectations of the patient and the therapist. Effective communication skills, including attentive listening and the use of clear understandable language, will improve the effectiveness of the therapist and lead to increased patient satisfaction and improved follow-through.[14] Martin and Tubbert[15] demonstrated an increase in patient follow-through in an exercise program when the person was involved in goal setting during program planning.

Conversely, the patient's contribution to goal setting may lack the precision or specificity necessary for adequate delineation of either the problem or the goal. Rogers and Figone[16] studied the life goals of persons with quadriplegia who were at least 1 year postdischarge. They found that most of their subjects were not following established goals and that they lacked the ability to develop goals for themselves.

Therapists can contribute to the formulation of a more adequate statement. The more global the statement of the problem, the less likely the goal will actually be achieved, given the short-term nature of the therapeutic process. Furthermore, there is less likelihood that there will be a clear awareness of achievement if it does occur or of how it was achieved. For example, a global statement such as "walking" would be improved in terms of the issues just described if a more specific statement were made such as "walking between parallel bars for 10 feet." Such a goal statement may be more short term and more easily measured by both the therapist and the patient. Both are more likely to see results and be therefore gratified. Thus a specific statement of the goal makes it more functional and enables a person to continue to provide effort in an ongoing way. The task of follow-through is made even more difficult when clients have chronic or complex conditions which may require rather lengthy or strenuous treatments.

Given the more typical understanding of the word "compliance," a patient may be considered to be "noncompliant" even with goals that he or she has set for himself/herself as well as with instructions given by a health professional. Nevertheless, the evidence briefly reviewed here suggests that patients who are more highly involved in the decision making are more likely to follow through on those decisions than are patients who are merely told what to do. We also realize that some patients are not capable, for various reasons, of taking an active role in their planning, even when essential facts have been clearly explained to them. In such cases, the health professional does what is legally and ethically best for the patient. In taking such a role, the health professional must understand the limited commitment thus made by the patient to his or her own care.

The process of therapy is considered to be an ongoing planning/evaluation system as described in Figure 1–1. A plan is made after an initial assessment, the plan is then implemented with evaluation going on integral to such implementation, and a new plan is made when indicated. The problem is how to enable the patient to take the maximal possible degree of participation in planning and then evaluation, and by so doing, to take an equivalent active role in the ongoing implementation of the plan—to commit the energy to make success more likely. The therapist must do everything possible to help the client assume responsibility, that is, to speak for oneself as a prerequisite

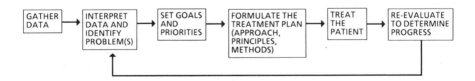

**FIGURE 1–1.** Treatment planning process. (From Trombly, CA: Occupational Therapy for Physical Dysfunction, ed 2. Williams & Wilkins, Baltimore, 1983, with permission.)

for acting for oneself. Thus one may optimize treatment outcomes and demonstrate the efficacy of treatments.

Issues of compliance, patient participation, and assumption of responsibility are not merely theoretical ones. A group of therapists in practice were asked about the relevance of these issues to their day-to-day work with clients. These therapists emphasized that they perceived patient participation to be at the core of the way health professionals seek to function. In recognition of these issues, the most recent revision of the Code of Ethics for Occupational Therapy emphasizes a concern for the welfare and dignity of the recipient of services. Among the criteria are that the persons served be included in the treatment-planning process and that goal-directed services be provided. Patient participation is thus now recognized to be essential to the delivery of good-quality care and is incorporated as a factor in the evaluation of rehabilitation facilities. Additionally, the need for patient participation could be a means of dealing with the important issue of staff "burnout."

The problem, then, that this book is designed to address is how to bring about more effective collaboration in planning between the patient and the therapist. The goals must arise from the patient to the maximal extent possible, consistent with making those goals clear, specific, and operational. It is the patient alone who can ultimately determine whether a goal is worth working for. It is the patient who must expend the energy if the goal is to be accomplished. Therefore, the core content of the goal must come from the patient and must be stated in terms that the patient can understand, as well as the therapist. If this is accomplished during the planning process, then the term "compliance" ceases to be appropriate. "Compliance" infers obedience to rules and regulations, to instructions given. It would be more useful to invite the person to become a collaborative partner to the extent possible. The therapist is thus operating at the level of making recommendations or offering suggestions rather than giving orders. Working with a therapeutic plan made by the patient then becomes an act of freedom and responsibility for the patient rather than one of obedience or compliance.

## WHAT ARE THE GOALS?

The goal of this book is integral to the overall goal of therapy and therapy schools which state that the student/clinician will be able to solve problems effectively. It is assumed that clinical problem solving is both internal and interactive. The internal aspect is concerned with the process that goes on in the health professional's head as he or she deals with the data provided in the clinical interview, in history taking, and in evaluation. From all these sources the clinician must determine both the impairments and the disabilities in order to develop an appropriate treatment plan including goals, means, and time line. All three of these comprise a plan. The determination of the patient's disabilities, the functional consequences of impairments, involves an interactive problem-solving process. This is the process by which one involves the patient from the start in the definition of the problem and decisions about goals. Eventually, one also involves the patient in the evaluation of outcomes and the efficacy of treatments and thus enables participation in all aspects of a plan. It is the interactive aspect of clinical problem solving that this book describes.

It is also important to say what this book does not attempt to do. It is not a complete textbook on communication with patients in the therapeutic setting. Although it may be considered in the context of psychosocial aspects of clinical practice, it is not a primer in patient counselling. It also does not attempt to be a textbook on clinical problem solving in occupational and physical therapy in all its aspects. For all these above topics, the interested reader is referred to other books.[17-19] This book is specifically one that describes a method for involving patients in self-directed management of those aspects of their lives affected by their disabilities. In so doing, it is likely that therapists will be dealing with an area of the patient's life that is crucial to the person's needs. In their area of professional competence both physical and occupational therapists will increase their ability to enable persons with disabilities to enhance their function and sense of self.

In summary, the overall objective of this book is that the student/clinician will be able to carry out the planning of a therapeutic regimen *with* a client and maintain patient participation throughout the therapeutic process, including ongoing evaluation of outcomes and means.

A plan includes (1) *goal(s)* (end, outcome, result) that is specific and relevant to the concern(s), (2) *means* (procedures, actions, methods), and (3) *time line* (due date by which the goal is to be accomplished and evaluated).

Enabling objectives include the following:

1. Determine the major concerns with maximal patient input.
2. Generate a specific goal statement in an area relevant to the patient's major concern with patient participation to the maximal extent possible.
3. Evaluate the goals initially set with maximum patient participation.
4. Revise goals and the time by which goals will be accomplished with maximal patient participation.
5. Specify the treatment procedures/equipment needs with maximum patient participation.

## APPLICATION TO ONESELF

The method by which the goals are to be achieved is that of experiential learning; that is, the instructor enables the student to function, just as the therapist will in turn enable the patient to function within the clinical setting. The student is involved in planning for his or her educational program

**TABLE 1 – 1.**

1. **What are my concerns about involving patients in the planning of their treatment?** List at least 3, and indicate which one you consider to be the most important by placing an asterisk next to it.

A.

B.

C.

**TABLE 1 – 2.**

1. **What are my concerns about involving patients in the planning of their treatment?** List at least 3, and indicate which one you consider to be the most important by placing an asterisk next to it.

A. Patients with cognitive deficits.

B. Patient unable to comprehend the questions asked.

C. Goals that are too general.*

**TABLE 1 – 3. (Group)**

1. **What are your concerns about involving patients in the planning of their treatment?**

A. Different levels of participation: e.g., patients who are depressed, want to be left alone; patients who use denial of any problem; unmotivated patients; different levels of cognitive function; problems in developing trust in a short time; the limits of patient versus professional responsibility.

B. Goals not in agreement: e.g., problems in communication; setting unrealistic goals; patient's goals not in agreement with those of professional; rapidly changing goals.

C. Follow-through of goals: e.g., carry over postdischarge, families unable to carry out goals due to lack of understanding; parents able to follow through as therapists interfering with the parental role.

or career development as an analogy for the type of activity the therapist will carry out with the patient. As described throughout, the instructor helps the student participate to the maximal degree in defining for oneself answers to the same questions that the therapist will in turn use with patients. The exercise presented in Table 1–1 marks the beginning of such participation. Table 1–2 illustrates the application of Table 1–1 by a student to herself. Table 1–3 is an example of a list of concerns generated by a group of practicing therapists. If you have difficulty in describing your own concerns, you may select from those listed by others.

# 2

# *Patient as Planner*

## WHAT ARE THE GOALS?

The previous chapter outlined the issues of defining goals so that they are relevant to the person's concerns or needs, and the importance of specifying those needs. This chapter will deal with the ways one can actually go about doing so with clients. The aim is to prepare the therapist to conduct an interview with a patient/client during which the second of the enabling objectives described in the entire process of developing a *plan* will be met. The aim is to generate a specific goal statement in an area relevant to the patient's major concern and with maximal patient participation. In order to accomplish this with the client, the therapist first meets those same goals in respect to his or her participation in the educational program.

## WHAT ARE THE PROBLEMS?

### IDENTIFYING NEEDS

The steps leading to the development of a treatment plan start with defining the problem. Only after the problem has been identified can one then set goals as one of the important parts of the total treatment plan which will also include the methods and the time line.[20]

In taking the history, it is common practice to ask the patient some version of the question "What brings you to therapy?" It is often identified in interview forms as "Chief Complaint." Although such information is sought from the patient and is frequently expressed in the patient's own words, the "actual" problem is defined by some sort of test or evaluation which is considered more objective and therefore more valid. When assessing a patient via the neurologic examination, muscle testing, joint range of motion, or grip strength, one is defining the existence of "impairments" such as paraplegia or muscle weakness of the knee extensors. The purpose of rehabilitation is frequently not to deal with the underlying impairments, which may remain stable. Rather, the purpose is to deal with the reorganization of the person (in regard to skills and attitudes) so that he or she can better deal with the functional consequences of such impairments—deal with "disabilities." It is the definition of the disabilities that requires input from the person; these functional consequences must be defined in the person's own terms.

For example, as a result of paraplegia a person may have difficulty getting around. Another example is that as a consequence of weakness of the knee extensors, an individual cannot stand in order to transfer from bed to chair. Or a stroke victim with a paralyzed upper extremity cannot cut meat or tie a shoe. It is the loss of mobility, the inability to transfer, or the inability to grasp a utensil or to pinch a shoelace that is the "disability." Furthermore, it is only the person with the problem who can define what is sometimes a very individualistic effect of an impairment—what may indeed be the highest priority in dealing with multiple disabilities.

It is important at this juncture to distinguish between different levels of thinking about human performance. Napier[13] described 3 different levels. The first is structural performance at the level of individual anatomic components, such as the knee joint. The second level of functional performance is the interaction between the various structural components to carry out an action, such as walking. At the third, or behavioral, level, the functional components are further combined to act in the context of a setting, such as work. Here an example might be being able to deliver the mail. The therapist must be sensitive to the fact that the patient, family, and the professionals involved may have concerns at multiple levels. For example, a person with a hand injury may need to deal with any or all of the following: (1) wound healing, (2) joint range of motion, (3) strength, (4) coordination, (5) work, (6) leisure, (7) social roles. Any single aspect may be more or less important at various times; priorities may shift.

The following example comes from a recent interview with a woman who has developed a left hemiplegia after the occlusion of one of the blood vessels of the brain:

**Therapist:** What are your concerns?
**Patient:** My left side is weak.
**Therapist:** What problems does the weakness of your left side cause you?
**Patient:** I have trouble going up and down steps.
**Therapist:** What sort of trouble do you have going up and down steps?
**Patient:** I'm afraid I will lose my balance on my steep front steps.

Only the patient can best determine, in the context of her own life setting, the specific aspects that are disabling about the impairment of her left side. Still another person with the same impairment may have quite a different life setting, with different consequences.

Similarly, when listing a number of areas of disability (such as mobility, transfers, and activities of daily living), all may be relevant to the person's future goals, but some may be of higher priority than others. For example, it may be less important for one person to take the time to learn to dress himself if he plans to have an attendant to help with this activity in order to be able to get to work on time.

The process of defining a problem is an ongoing one like any of the other aspects of the evaluation/planning process. The answers to the question regarding concerns will, of course, vary with the individual's degree of impairment, type of impairment, and the very individualistic setting in which the person needs to function. It is important also to recognize that the problem statement made by the client may change over time as thoughts become clearer, as problems are solved and new problems appear, and as one may feel more trust in the person who is asking. The ability to answer this or any other question also depends upon the skill of the patient in verbalizing what he or she is thinking or feeling. It is the task of the therapist to enable the patient to answer this question as freely and as fully as possible, recognizing the possibility of limited success at any one time.

In establishing what may be the "real" problem at any one time, it is useful to explore at least three times, by repeating the question as to concerns, before determining with the patient the highest priority problem or the clearest statement of the problem. Threefold exploration is a useful minimum but may not be sufficient to define the problem adequately. The ongoing quality of the therapist/client relationship permits re-exploration at any time. One may explore in depth, as in the case of the woman with the left-sided weakness wherein the questions were asked in a successive way by incorporating the answer previously given. One may describe that process exploration as "in depth."

Alternatively, one may explore "in breadth," as in the following example:

**Therapist:** What bothers you?
**Patient:** I have a tingling in my left side.
**Therapist:** Is there anything else bothering you?
**Patient:** I have trouble using my left ankle.
**Therapist:** Is there anything else?
**Patient:** I can't move my toes.
**Therapist:** What bothers you the most?
**Patient:** It's hard for me to walk.

It is the last statement that can then become the basis for generating a goal statement. After exploring these several alternatives and then making a selection, the likelihood is greater that the eventual goal will actually be relevant to the patient's needs.

In the next example of a student's interview of a person with a spinal cord injury, three concerns were generated. As is frequently the case, it is the third concern that is selected as most important:

**Therapist:** What are your concerns?
**Patient:** Dressing.
**Therapist:** Anything else?
**Patient:** Driving.
**Therapist:** Anything else?
**Patient:** Attendant care. Having a good attendant.
**Therapist:** What is your major concern?
**Patient:** Attendant care.

In the examples thus far, we have illustrated asking the patient to simply select the most important concern. One may also ask the patient to prioritize the concerns as first, second, and third in rank order. Still another option is to ask the patient to weight the concerns. The use of shared weights can permit a later rough quantification of resource allocation in reference to the priorities. The shared weighting procedure is done in the following manner: For example, in the case of 3 concerns, one compares the items within each pair such as A and B; A and C; then B and C. Three points are to be shared between each pair. One may assign 3 points to A and none to B; or 2 to A and 1 to B, and so forth. One would then sum the weights for each item to determine the final order. The following example was done with a patient by a student in occupational therapy.

## 1. What Are Your Concerns?

3 2      A. I can't drive and get around.   (5)
0   1     B. I don't have many outside interests.   (1)
  1 2    C. I can't propel my wheelchair very far.   (3)

In this example, 5 points were assigned to the first item, and 3 points to the third item, whereas the second item had less weight. One can thus later make a rough allocation of resources to the various items with $5/9$ to the highest priority item, $3/9$ to the second, and $1/9$ to the third.

It is noteworthy to realize that there are different bases for attaching priorities to any item. Therapists during an in-service training program identified several different reasons: the frequency of the problem, the severity or intensity of the problem, the one that would be most difficult to overcome, and the one that is the easiest to overcome.

In order to evaluate the degree to which the patient has adequately explored his or her concerns and properly identified what is the major concern, one may use a "check-out" procedure. The selected statement can be fed back for the patient to agree to. It is also sometimes useful to go a step further in this process by asking the patient to state what he or she has agreed to and thus "confirm" what is the statement of the "real" concern. One may use a statement such as "I would like to make sure we are both on the same wavelength by your telling me what you have just now agreed to." This extra step of confirmation is usually used when there has been some difficulty on the part of the therapist in clearly understanding what is being said or when the patient seems unsure. It is important to emphasize that the entire process of exploration and selection is nonjudgmental; that is, the therapist does not approve or disapprove of the statements made by the patient. One seeks to elicit the patient's concerns and priorities. At a later time, one may need to arrive at a cooperative agreement if there are differences between the therapist and the patient.

The following is an example of an interview of a hospitalized patient carried out by a therapy student.

1. **What Are Your Concerns?**
    A. I can't play golf because of pain in my hand when I hold the club.
    B. I can't spread mayonnaise, open a jar, or open a milk carton by myself.
    C. I can't get dressed and put my socks on without help from my wife.
2. **What Is Your Greatest Concern?**
    I can't put my socks on by myself.
3. **Check out:**  agreed    confirmed

The time spent initially in the process of defining a problem is generally well spent. In one recent interview, a person with amputation of both lower extremities of many years' duration was asked about her concerns now that she had a new, second set of prostheses. In the process of the threefold exploration of concerns, she was able to describe to a therapist for the first time what she later said had troubled her for the past 10 years. She stated that she had always been concerned about injuring herself if she fell because she had never been taught how to fall and get up again without injury. No one had offered her the chance before to express what she really felt she needed. On the basis of this process of exploration, she established as a high priority in her therapy program learning how to get up from the floor and then learning how to fall without hurting herself.

Now that one has explored concerns and made some judgment as to priorities in the selection step, the next task is to specify the problem. For example, the statement "my shoulder hurts" merely answers the question as the *what* the problem may be. A more specific statement would be "my left shoulder hurts at night to the degree that I can't sleep." Such a statement answers not only *what* but *where* and *when* and *how much*. It is generally useful to specify the chief complaint so that it meets at least a 3-point criterion of answering not only *what* but either *where* or *when* in terms of the setting and either *how much* or *how long* or some other measure addressing *to what degree*. Problems dealing with the issue of specification will be described more fully in the next section in conjunction with the specification of the goal statement.

## SPECIFYING GOALS

The aim is to generate a "specific" goal statement in an area relevant to the patient's main concern with maximal patient participation. In the previous section we looked at the process of identifying the major concern. Once the problem has been identified and defined, the next step is to establish goals that, when accomplished, would indicate that the problem has been alleviated. The goal statement describes the outcome, that is, the results that one seeks to have happen. The goal should be relevant to the patient's main concern. For example, if the main concern was an inability to dress myself, then one obvious goal could be "to be able to put on a shirt."

One concern listed in the previous section was "pain in the left shoulder at night so that I can't sleep." Evidence that the problem is being solved would be a goal statement relevant to the main concern, which could vary depending on the person who is experiencing the pain. One such goal statement could be "I will be able to get my usual 8 hours of sleep." Another might be "not have the pain interfere with my sleep." Still another option might be "my shoulder pain goes away."

Another person with a recent spinal cord injury (SCI) was concerned about the pain in his legs below the level of his injury. When he was asked to explore his concerns, he identified that his major concern was what the pain meant. His goal was to find out whether the feeling of pain meant that something was wrong that he needed to deal with. He met his goal when he was reassured that pain in persons with SCI below the level of their lesion did not necessarily signify that something serious was going on, as it may have prior to his injury. One cannot presuppose what a person's goal may be. One cannot assume that because one has pain the goal will always be a reduction of pain. It is necessary to ask about one's goals.

As with the question of concerns, one explores a minimum of three possible goals before selecting one as the highest priority, which is then described in greater detail (i.e., specified). (Of course, it is possible to start with more than one goal, but for purposes of illustration, we will deal with one in this instance.) One value of the exploration of goals is in dealing with the concern of some therapists that patients will set "unrealistic" goals when they are permitted to take a more active role in planning their therapy. If the patient initially mentions a goal that would require a longer-term commitment than is usually available to patients in the service setting, it is useful to ask the patient to consider shorter-term goals as part of the exploration process. The question can be phrased: "What might be the first step in meeting your goal?" It is important to enable patients to keep what might appear to another person to be an impossible dream while still defining some intermediate stage that would indicate progress.

The exploration step is also useful in dealing with the need to define the problem in functional terms rather than in terms of impairments, which may not be possible to overcome. As an example, one woman stated her concern: "I can't use my left arm." Her first goal statement dealt with regaining strength in her hand. When the therapist started to explore further goals, he prefaced the question by saying, "All people are different; the trouble with one's hand may mean different things, depending on what is really important to that person. What sorts of things would you like to be able to do that would make you feel that you are doing better?" Rather than limiting herself to goals relating to alleviating the impaired left arm, she now defined her disability in terms of taking care of her children. She eventually set one of her specific goals to be "fixing a grilled cheese sandwich at home for my children." With this more functional goal in mind, several different means by which she could accomplish it came to mind. Regaining strength in the hand is only one of several means, including technical aids, by which one can fix an acceptable grilled cheese sandwich.

Many therapists have difficulty distinguishing between *goals* and *means*. The *goal* statement relates to the outcomes, the results, the ends of the therapeutic intervention. Many persons enter into rehabilitation because of a loss of ways by which they have ordinarily carried out life's activities. What they ultimately seek to regain is the functional results—to be able to get around, to care for their bodily needs, to get sustenance. One is seeking a functional outcome, one that translates into life situations. It is often necessary to use alternative *means* to reach the goals. The goals frequently remain the same as prior to the injury; the means more often may need to change.

In the example of the woman with the weak left hand, she naturally originally focused on the loss of strength in her hand, but that is only a means to her ultimate functional goal of caring for her children. One essentially asked her *"why?"* in relation to her initial goal of strengthening her hand in order to help her move toward describing the more functional outcomes sought. The change in focus toward caring for her children is an important step in the process of rehabilitation which requires an acceptance of the possibility of alternatives, of ways of doing things that may be different from those used before. Goals such as increased range of motion and increased strength can be measurable and may be eminently desirable, yet they are only means to the more functional goals which are ultimately the basis upon which the therapeutic intervention must be judged. The threefold exploration step is an opportunity to aid this major change in thinking.

The exploration step can also be useful in leading the patient to think through goals more fully so that the first thing that comes to mind is not automatically accepted. One young man with a recent spinal cord injury initially stated his goal "to be like I was before my injury." As he further explored his goals, his next statement was "to be an athlete the way I was before." His final statement was "to understand the extent of my injuries and how they affect my future." Such exploration increases the possibility of some goals that can be shared by both the therapist and the client.

Just as the chief complaint could be selected, prioritized, or determined by a weighting system, so, too, the primary or first-order goal statement can be derived by any of these procedures. It is this first-order or short-term goal that can be specified.

The statement of the goal must be specific in order for it to be measurable. If it is measurable, it will be easier to demonstrate achievement. Thus far, in the exploration and selection steps, the goal statement merely helps answer the question of *"what?"* In order to meet the minimum criteria of adequate specificity, it is also necessary to answer the questions of *"where?"* and *"when?"* dealing with the setting in which the goal is to be accomplished. The setting in time in which the outcome is to be demonstrated can be an interview, the therapy session, and so forth. (The time line, the duration of the time before the goal is to be reached, is a separate item in the total *plan.*) The third question to be answered in defining a specific goal statement is some measure as to degree, such as *"how much?"* or *"how far?"*

Examples of specific goal statements are:

**What?** Generate a goal statement
**When?** in an interview
**How Well?** to meet the 3-point criterion of specificity.

**What?** Walk
**How Much?** for two feet
**Where?** between parallel bars
**When?** during my therapy session.

**What?** Turn over from side to side
**Where?** in the hospital bed
**How Often?** every 3 hours.

## PATIENT PARTICIPATION

The aim thus far has been to generate a specific goal statement in an area relevant to the patient's main concern, with "maximal patient participation." We have looked at the use of the two basic questions of concerns and goals; their relationship to each other; and the steps of exploration, selection, and specification to be used in answering them. The third major aspect is the degree to which the answers arise from the patient as opposed to from the therapist. It has been our assumption in dealing with the problem of patient commitment to carrying out the therapy that participation in the planning will increase the degree to which effort will be available for the implementation of any program. The objective of "maximal" patient participation does not require any absolute level of participation; rather, it seeks to achieve the highest level of participation consistent with accomplishing the other objectives of identifying needs and specifying goals.

Table 2–1 describes the levels of participation in order of degree of involvement in the answering of the questions in carrying out the threefold exploration, selection, and specification.

The criteria for "maximal" patient participation includes starting the interview process with an open-ended question and moving down the levels of participation only one step at a time as necessary to meet the other objectives. Whenever possible, the interviewer should return to open-ended questions during the course of the interaction and should seek patient agreement to any change in the level of participation being used as well as to steps of exploration, selection, and specification.

To the extent possible, therefore, the therapist seeks to encourage the greatest possible patient participation by asking open-ended questions, enabling the person to function at the level of *free choice*. If, in order to meet the other aim of several answers in the exploration step or in meeting the aims of a specific goal statement the therapist needs to begin to offer options, one would offer 3 suggestions, enabling the patient to function at *multiple choice*. The use of this level of participation should be prefaced by asking the agreement of the client: "Is it OK with you if I offer you some suggestions?" In the exploration step, it is frequently necessary to offer suggestions at some point which then serves to help the patient begin to state freely some of his own answers. It is usually necessary to use no lower level of participation than "multiple choice" in dealing with the exploration, selection, and specification of concerns and goals. There are obvious exceptions in that persons with cog-

| TABLE 2–1. Definitions of Levels of Patient Participation | | |
|---|---|---|
| **Therapist** | **Patient** | **Degree or Level** |
| Asks open-ended questions. (Does not suggest answers) | Free choice | A |
| Asks questions *and* offers suggestions (3 options). | Multiple choice | B |
| Asks questions *and* offers an answer-recommendation. | Forced choice Concurrence | C |
| Prescribes, does not ask; tells what to do. | No choice Compliant or noncompliant | D |

nitive difficulties and communication problems may require a lower level of participation. Maximal level of participation is merely defined as the highest level of participation consistent with meeting the other goals of the interactive planning process.

If it is necessary, one can then move to the next level of making a single recommendation so that the patient is acting at the level of *forced choice*. In this level of involvement, the options are not merely identified but the selection is already made in each instance, as to which answer would be best. This step should be prefaced by seeking agreement: "Is it OK with you if I give you a recommendation?"

It should not be necessary when dealing with concerns and goals to prescribe for the patient *(no choice)*. When the therapist acts to prescribe in terms of concerns and goals, the likelihood of commitment of energy to the treatment program has been lessened very severely. If it becomes necessary to do so, one may preface this last step in degree of involvement by seeking agreement: "Is it OK with you if I tell you what to do?" In general, the asking of the patient's permission to move down these various degrees of participation not only offers him or her the opportunity to accept or to reject the offer but also makes the therapist conscious of the changes in degree of control being carried out. It is this consciousness that is sought in the training program for the therapists, and the statements made to the patient offer confirmation that the therapist is aware of the changes being carried out.

It is surprising to many professionals how well patients do in generating their own goals when given the opportunity to do so. It is sometimes difficult for therapists to give the patient enough time to do this. Each therapist must develop his or her own level of tolerance for personal anxiety before intervening by "moving down the scale" in offering suggestions and thus taking a greater role for planning than may be necessary. As one moves down the scale, the more the goals arise from the therapist, the less commitment one may expect from the patient in achieving the goals. The therapist is legally and ethically responsible for insuring that the goals are scientifically relevant to the patient's impairment as well as relevant to the patient's concerns. The exploration step in eliciting at least 3 answers to the planning questions makes it likely that at least one of the concerns and goals is mutually compatible to both the therapist and the patient.

## APPLICATION TO ONESELF

In the exercise at the end of Chapter 1, you were asked to explore the first question as to concerns and to make a selection of your area of greatest concern. That exercise marked the start of your participation in learning how to use this approach by doing it for yourself. At this point, having reviewed Chapter 2, your concerns may be somewhat different from those you originally considered. Your answers may change as you encounter new dimensions of the process of learning to involve patients in a meaningful way in their own program planning. At this time, therefore, you should once again explore your concerns and make a selection. The exploration step can go on in depth if there is but one problem initially identified. You can then successively ask the question as to "what is troublesome about _____ [whatever the expressed concern was]?" You can also explore by listing several problems, asking "What else do I find difficult about learning how to involve patients in their own planning?" Use Table 2–2 as an exercise to begin this reexamination of your concerns relative to this course.

As described earlier in this chapter, the selection process may involve shared weights or simple prioritization. Once you have made a selection of the best statement of concern or the most important problem, you should then "check out" or "confirm" the validity of the selection: "Is this what really bothers me the most?"

You may go on in the exercise to explore your personal goals in this course by listing 3 successive steps or 3 alternative goals. Then identify the major goal or the one that you want to accomplish first. These are your goals for yourself in learning the content of this course. The final goal statement should be specified, as described earlier in this chapter.

It is important to emphasize once again the distinction to be made between goals and means. For example, a student, when asked to state a goal for himself, mentioned "jogging 5 miles a day 3 days each week." Although this may be a desirable action and one that is measurable, the statement does not define the functional outcome he sought to achieve. It is comparable to many goals set in therapy that are really activities or means. It is helpful to ask *why* one is choosing to jog. In this case, the possible outcomes may include weight reduction, increased oxygen efficiency, decreased heart rate, and so forth. One could ask the question *why* once again and go to another level of outcome, which might be expressed in terms of increased longevity, reduced incidence of heart disease, and so forth. Once his goal has been identified, he can consider possible alternative means by which such a health improvement program could be achieved. Jogging is only one of many means for doing so. One can go on even further to define the outcomes in terms of *why* one would be interested in living longer. However, three-fold exploration provides a reasonable limit for such activity.

The rehabilitation planning process frequently requires the patient to clarify the distinction between the ends and the means in order to continue to achieve one's life goals despite the loss of some of the previously used means. In order to help patients make this distinction, the student/therapist must be able to do so for himself or herself first; one cannot give away what one does not have. In this exercise, as in the clinical setting, it is essential to define the goals or outcomes sought before considering the alternative means for achieving those outcomes. A therapist is trained to offer methods for treatment, but these decisions must be deferred until one has adequately identified the outcomes; that is, goals must be defined before means can be rationally selected.

TABLE 2-2. **Program Planning Sheet 1 (PPS-1)**

Patient _____  Date _____
                                            Therapist _____

PROGRAM PLANNING SHEET 1

1. What are your concerns?
   A.
   B.
   C.

2. What is your greatest concern?
   Check out: _____ agreed _____ confirmed

3. What do you want to see happen? What would make you feel that
   you are making progress in dealing with your chief concern? What
   are your goals?
   A.
   B.
   C.

4. What is your specific goal?
   A   B   C   D      What?
   A   B   C   D      Setting?
   A   B   C   D      Degree?

5. Please circle the "lowest" level of participation used in answer to
   the various portions of the goal statement.
   A = open-ended question: FREE CHOICE
   B = suggestions (3 options): MULTIPLE CHOICE
   C = recommendation (1 option): FORCED CHOICE
   D = Prescription (tell what to do): NO CHOICE

Still another issue that has been difficult for many therapists is *personalization* of the concerns and goals. Personalizing is achieved by the use of personal pronouns in defining concerns and goals that are one's own. It is a matter of clearly articulating ownership of the concerns and goals; for example, "I am concerned that _____ ." "I would like to _____ ." For example, one therapist said "I am concerned about my ability to help patients set "realistic" goals," the therapist's specific goal might be "During my next interview, I would like to see the patient describe 3 goals, to the degree that they are consistent with what 50% of persons with the same degree of neurologic involvement are able to achieve." Another therapist who had a similar concern stated her goal as "The patient will ambulate independently on the ward for 60 feet." This latter goal did not deal with *her* concern about her skill in enabling the patient to set realistic goals.

If you have not already done so, complete the exercise using Table 2-2. If you have trouble understanding how to apply the steps in the exercise to yourself, there are several examples of how other students have completed this same exercise for themselves in Tables 2-3 and 2-4. However, work as independently as possible without recourse to these examples until after you have made some effort to arrive at your own responses.

Program planning sheet 1 (PPS-1) is one version of the form that is used with patients. Note that the level of participation is important when you use it for patients. When you use it for yourself, you do not need to consider the level of participation in specifying the goal. As we go along, this basic form will change as more questions are added for you to use for yourself and with patients. Each line of specification is scored separately; when this is transferred to the medical record, only the lowest level of patient participation need be stated. If you choose to do weighting of your concerns, draw a small chart for that purpose in the right or left hand margin of the form, as illustrated in Table 2-4.

## APPLICATION TO PATIENT CARE

Having had the opportunity to become familiar with the process for oneself, the therapist can now help the patient do so for himself or herself. Use PPS-1 (found in Table 2-2) to interview several people—including patients, if that is possible in your circumstances.

You will use the form with patients or others differently from the way you used it for yourself because the form reflects the degree of patient participation in eliciting the answers to the segments of the goal statement. The first step, after introducing yourself and stating the general purpose of the interview, is to explore concerns with the patient. Some students have had difficulty in asking the question regarding concerns in ways that are directly applicable to a patient. For example, a patient first described his concern as not

---

**TABLE 2-3. Example of Student Use of Concerns and Goals Sections of the Form.**

Patient _____    Date _____
                                         Therapist _____

PROGRAM PLANNING SHEET 1

1. What are your concerns?
   A. I am concerned about integrating this system smoothly into a patient interview.
   B. Will I be able to get the patient to see the difference between goals and means?
   *C. Can I get the patient to "open up" and share his concerns and goals with me?

2. What is your greatest concern?
   Will I be able to get the patient to "open up' and share his concerns and goals with me?

Check out: ___*_*___ agreed _____ confirmed

3. What do you want to see happen? What would make you feel that you are making progress? What are your goals?
   A. I will feel comfortable in the interview.
   *B. I will get a clear statement of concerns and goals from the patient.
   C. The patient will talk freely to me.

4. What is your specific goal?
   What:      I will complete Form 1
   Setting:   During a 20-minute patient interview
   Degree:    To the extent that I elicit 3 concerns, a chief concern, 3 goals, and 1 specific goal.

---

being able to walk. When he denied any other concerns, the next question in exploring concerns could have been: "What might be keeping you from walking?" rather than giving up on concerns at that point.

Do all of the things that have been discussed in this chapter: Explore several concerns in depth or breadth; have the patient select one chief concern (either by weighting or by simply selecting the greatest concern); explore several goals that would progress the patient toward alleviating that concern; have the patient select the greatest concern and specify it. Table 2–5 may be used by both student and instructor to evaluate the *process* or sequential progression of the interview with the inclusion of all components we recommend. Examples of student interviews of patients may be found in Tables 2–6, 2–7, and 2–8.

One important stimulus to the process of patient participation is providing evidence that the patient's statements are being heard. One very useful

**TABLE 2-4. Example of Use of Weighting to Select Main Concern; Use of Form PPS-1 by Student for Her Own Concerns**

Patient _____  Date _____
                                   Therapist _____

PROGRAM PLANNING SHEET 1

1. What are your concerns?
   3    2    = 5    A. I am concerned that I won't be able to use this method with aphasic patients.
   0         1 = 1  B. I'm afraid that I won't remember the questions when I get to the interview.
        1    2 = 3  C. I am concerned that I won't be able to think of multiple-choice options when I need them.

2. What is your greatest concern?
   I am concerned that I won't be able to use this method with aphasic patients
   during an interview in clinic
   to the degree that I will be able to elicit patient concerns and goals

Check out: ___X___ agreed _____ confirmed

3. What would you like to see happen that would make you feel that you were making progress with your chief concern?
   A. I will develop a nonverbal communication system with the patient (e.g., head nodding).
   B. I will feel comfortable talking to an aphasic person.
   C. I will establish an aphasic patient's concerns and goals.

4. What is your first goal?
   What:    I will communicate with an aphasic patient using nonverbal communications
   Setting: in an interview in clinic
   Degree:  to the degree that I will have a chief complaint and goal statement which the patient agrees to by nodding.

technique for doing this is to record patient statements on a pad of paper in full view of the patient, repeating aloud what you are writing as you write it. This provides very direct evidence that the patient is being heard. This procedure also provides a record of the interview for later analysis and discussion with students or colleagues. Table 2–6 is a straightforward application of the process as discussed in this chapter. Table 2–7 illustrates a more flexible use of the process; 6 concerns are elicited, 3 are first selected by asking the patient to narrow the list to 3, than 1 of the 3 is chosen by the patient as his or her chief concern.

**TABLE 2–5. Interview Evaluation Form: Patient Participation in Planning for Therapy**

| | Not Attempted | Attempted | | Comments |
|---|---|---|---|---|
| | | Incomplete | Complete | |
| 1. Did interviewer<br>　A. introduce patient to overall procedures?<br>　B. introduce exploration of concerns?<br>　C. elicit at least 3 concerns?<br>　D. ask for selection of priorities (either shared weights or priority)?<br>　E. confirm major concern(s)?<br>　F. introduce exploration of goals?<br>　G. introduce cooperative role in identifying goals?<br>　H. elicit 3 goals?<br>　I. ask for selection of one goal to pursue?<br>　J. specify goal:　what?<br>　K. 　　　　　　　　setting?<br>　L. 　　　　　　　　degree?<br>2. Did interview start with open-ended question?<br>3. Did interviewer ask patient's consent before moving to multiple choice, forced choice, or prescription?<br>4. Did student move down steps in correct order?<br>5. Did student return to open-ended questions at an appropriate time? | | | | |

---

**TABLE 2-6.  Example of Use of PPS-1 with a Patient, by a Student, Sections on Concerns and Goals**

Patient _____  Date _____
                                            Therapist _____

PROGRAM PLANNING SHEET 1

1. What are your concerns?
   A. I cannot play golf once a week with my friends like I did a year ago because holding a golf club in my hand is painful.
   B. I cannot spread mayonnaise on bread, open a jar or milk carton when I want to eat, without someone helping me.
   *C. I cannot get dressed without help from my wife.

2. What is your greatest concern?
   I can't get dressed by myself.

3. Check out: ___*_*___ agreed _____ confirmed

4. What do you want to see happen? What would make you feel that you are making progress in relation to your major concern? What are your goals?
   A. I want to be able to put on my socks by myself.
   B. I want to be able to put on my pants by myself.
   *C. I want to be able to put on my shirt without help.

5. What is your specific goal?
   (A)  B   C   D   What:     put on my shirt
   (A)  B   C   D   Setting:  in the morning
   A   (B)  C   D   Degree:   in less than 10 minutes and without help

---

Table 2–8 presents the most complete interview and deserves more comment. It concerns a 41-year-old female hairdresser who sustained a near amputation of the left upper extremity (LUE) above the elbow with fracture at the junction of the distal and middle third of the humerus. She was initially seen by a hand therapist at bedside for fabrication of a volar static wrist splint. She was wearing a humeral external fixator at the time of the interview. Whenever she did not understand a question, she asked the therapist to give her examples. She did not use the examples for her answers and was very verbal during the interview.

Note that the therapist elicited more than 3 concerns, then selected 3 and weighted them to get the chief complaint. This also illustrates the flexibility of the system.

One aspect of patient participation is to state clearly to the patient the goals for the interview and the steps for reaching those goals. As one student put it, it helps to let the patient in on what you are doing as you do it. You start by telling the patient that you are going to explore what might be prob-

---

**TABLE 2-7. Example of a Student Interview with a Patient using PPS-1 as a Guide**

Patient _____ Date _____
Therapist _____

1. What are your concerns?
   A. dressing
   B. driving
   C. attendant care—hiring a good attendant
   D. cooking
   E. fishing and hunting
   F. working a computer fully

2. What are your major concerns?
   A. dressing
   *B. attendant care
   C. working the computer

3. What would you like to see happen in relation to your major concern; what would make you feel that you were making progress?
   A. knowing that someone is trustworthy and will have time to help with shopping
   B. finding an attendant I can get along with
   *C. find an attendant

4. What is your first goal?
   Ⓐ  B   C   D      What:      Find an attendant
   A   B   Ⓒ   D      Setting:   to be with me at home
   A   B   Ⓒ   D      Degree:    with whom I would feel confident doing hands-on care.

---

lems. Then you ask the patient what would make him or her feel that there had been some progress in dealing with those problems. The ground rules are further described in terms of hearing from the patient what he or she is concerned about and what might be some goals for him or her. You may tell the patient at the beginning that you will help if he or she "gets stuck" but that it is important for the patient to tell you what matters to him or her. Some patients may be surprised to be involved in goal setting, thinking it to be the therapist's responsibility. In such a case, you should convey to the patient the reasons for inviting such participation as expressed throughout this book.

There are 2 aspects to the interview. One is the answers that are documented on the form and that can later be used for writing notes in the medical record. The other aspect is the process or method by which the answers are generated. The "level of participation" is an important part of this latter aspect. It can tell you how much the answers on the form are the patient's, and thus their strength or value in planning. Be aware of the level of participation as the interview progresses. Each time you feel you need to change the

---

**TABLE 2-8. Example of an Interview Done by an Occupational Therapist**

Patient _____  Date _____8-5-88_____
                                    Therapist _____

1. What are your concerns?
   A. being able to dress myself
   B. like to know if I can return to hair dressing if I want
   C. can I grasp a glass? can I grasp things with my fingers?
   D. will I become depressed?
   E. will the pain continue or subside?
   F. could the arm eventually "flare up" (e.g., arthritis)?
   G. afraid to drive at night

2. What are your major concerns?
   0         0 = 0A. mental attitude
        0    3 = 3B. arm flare-up
   3    3       = 6C. pain
   Pain confirmed as chief concern.

3. What are your goals?
   *A. that I could go to sleep at night and sleep well without drugs
   B. that I could tolerate pain for longer periods of time (e.g., while I grip a broom and sweep the kitchen floor or while ironing)*
   C. that I could tolerate massage of my fingers (e.g., tolerate force of shower water on my hand)*

4. What is your first goal?
   Ⓐ  B  C  D    What:    a good night's rest
   Ⓐ  B  C  D    Setting: at home
   A  Ⓑ  C  D    Degree:  straight through without disturbance from my fingers

---

*Examples were elicited when I asked her for functional examples.

level of participation, notify the patient of the change and seek his or her agreement to that change before proceeding, for example, "Is it OK if I give you some suggestions?" This respects the patient's dignity and alerts your instructor that you know what is happening in the interview.

The final component of Form PPS–1 is the recording of the level of patient participation in the development of each aspect of the specified goal. Simply circle A, B, C, or D to indicate *the lowest* level of patient participation needed in the final specification of the goal. This level of participation may be important in evaluating the outcomes of the *plan* at a later date (see Chapter 3). It is, therefore, useful to document the lowest level of participation necessary in order to specify the goal. In later chapters we also change the A B C D format to a simple line that asks for level of participation. After you learn the system, it can be used flexibly.

If it is necessary to move to "multiple choice," then the goal statement is scored at that level of participation, even if only 1 portion of the goal statement required that degree of therapist contribution. Students sometimes have difficulty thinking of multiple-choice options—in fact, experienced therapists sometimes have the same difficulty. Experience with a variety of patients partially alleviates this problem; still, the third option is sometimes a rather weak "or something else." Sometimes options can be found in the sequence of an activity, (e.g., stand, balance, walk). At other times the memory of what other patients with similar problems have done will give you cues to options. Sometimes degrees (e.g., mild, moderate, or severe pain) will provide ideas for options. With practice, your skill will grow.

An intermediate step that has often proven helpful to students is to ask friends if they would allow you to interview them. Start by asking, "Do you have any problems or concerns right now that you would be willing to share with me?" Try to keep it "real" and avoid role playing. Role playing can be a very effective learning tool in a controlled environment where everyone knows exactly what is occurring, but we recommend that you keep your interviews as grounded in reality as possible. Students have proven quite creative in finding opportunities to practice interviewing and have reported some interesting experiences in class.

# 3

# *Patient as Evaluator*

## WHAT ARE THE GOALS?

The previous chapter was concerned with improving patient participation in the implementation of treatment plans by increasing both the specificity of the goals and their relevance to patient concerns. The addition of the question as to outcomes in this chapter now completes one cycle of the ongoing planning process. One may then revise the concerns and goals including revision of the time prior to the next evaluation. The aim is to enable the patient to participate in this evaluation and ongoing revision to the maximal degree possible.

## WHAT ARE THE PROBLEMS?

### EVALUATING OUTCOMES

One concern of therapists is the maintenance of commitment by patients with chronic impairments to perform what may be strenuous activities, particularly when such activities need to go on over a rather long period of time. To a lesser extent, commitment may also be a problem for more short-time patients. What has been thus far accomplished in setting an initial goal with the patient is but a necessary first step in dealing with this problem. The need to maintain enthusiasm is not limited to the patient but also applies to staff to prevent "burnout." One must see results, and those results must somehow be connected to what was being sought. The need for documentation of results is also increasingly required by third-party payers as well as accreditation agencies.

The initial specification of the goal statement in terms understandable to both the therapist and the patient permits evaluation of outcomes to take place. Our emphasis on patient participation in defining outcomes as well as goals is, as far as we know, unique in the literature. Our experience supports the usefulness of inviting such participation. Therapy or rehabilitation may be seen as a recurrent planning cycle. The process includes the making of plan(s) after an initial assessment, implementation of the plan, evaluation integral to such implementation, and revision of the plan in light of experience in an ongoing cycle. Patient participation in the evaluation and ongoing revision of plans can be expected to contribute to a greater degree of participation in a treatment program that is also ongoing. The long-term commitment of the patient to his or her care is enhanced if he or she is taught during therapy to be observant of the outcomes of efforts to meet goals.

This process of evaluation now leads us to the third question to be used in planning with the patient: *What has been accomplished in relation to the goal?* It is important to review the goals initially established and to relate this new question to the previous plan. The same 3 steps are used in answering this question as used with the first 2 questions, that is, exploration, selection, and specification. As one therapist expressed it, "The patient hearing himself describe some positive outcomes helps the person feel better about what has been happening. It helps the patient to keep putting out the effort necessary." Since that is the aim, the exploration of at least three aspects of any outcome or several different outcomes reinforces the sense that something positive did occur. To achieve this effect, the statements in regard to accomplishments should arise from the patient to the maximal extent possible. Just as in answering the questions as to concerns and goals, the therapist should start with open questions ("free choice"), and go down the scale of participation a step at a time as needed after asking the patient's permission to do so.

The exploration of what outcomes were achieved may require a greater awareness of some of the intermediate outcomes than there may have been when setting the original sequence of goals. One may find that there are many more small incremental steps to go through. If one focuses on these smaller steps that one has accomplished, there is a greater sense of success than when one focuses only on the larger, more global goals. It is important to recognize those outcomes which are achieved, even if they are but a partial accomplishment of the original set of goals. There may have been somewhat smaller increments than initially envisaged. Alternatively, larger or unanticipated accomplishments may have occurred.

The subsequent selection step can be based upon either of the techniques for selection illustrated in relation to concerns and goals. A paired weighting technique may be used, or one may determine what was the result about which the person felt the best or recalls the best. The value of making a selection lies mainly in focusing the patient on a scene that he or she can then more readily relive. A major objective of this question is to enable the person to savor and to take credit for the accomplishments, rather than to report one's failures and perhaps then to take blame for them, which is the more common experience.

The specification of the selected outcome should describe not only *what* was accomplished but both *when* and *where*. It is particularly useful for the person to visualize the setting to the maximal degree possible. It is in recollection of that scene that the person may be more likely to relive and savor the experience. In the context of that scene, the person may then be better able to consider the possible actions that may have contributed to the outcome. Criteria of specificity would also include some quantitative measure, such as *How much?* or *How far?* An example of such a specific statement of outcome would be "I just now walked 5 feet in my room."

## REVISION OF GOALS AND TIME LINE

The addition of the question as to outcome will now permit the patient to participate in the making of a revised set of goals in the ongoing therapeutic process. As the therapist and the patient explore together the results that have been achieved, the patient may become even more active in once again addressing the question of concerns and new goals, revised in the light of experience.

Thus far the client/patient has been a participant in defining problems and then goals relevant to those concerns as a major component of a more total *plan*. We have emphasized that the *plan* includes at least two items in addition to the goal. One of these other components is the means or methods by which the goals are to be accomplished. The participation of the client in helping define that important aspect will be described in the next chapter. Still another component is the time line. The time line defines the duration of the *plan;* operationally, it is the time when one will again evaluate outcome. Until now, the issue of patient participation in helping define this aspect has been deferred. In many instances, addressing the question of outcome permits a more effective appraisal by both the therapist and the patient of the rate of progress that may be expected. The patient may now more effectively participate in the revision not only of the problem and the goal but also of the time line to be set for the next cycle of evaluation.

One is making explicit the principle of cyclicity, a procedure that permits progression from initial concern to final discharge. Concerns change as previous goals are met and new issues arise; or as previous goals are attempted and the reality of outcomes are faced. Outcomes stimulate reassessment and redefinition of problems and goals and the time that may be required to accomplish them, in life as well as in therapy.

# INTEGRATION INTO THE CLINICAL RECORD

The third issue is the integration of this approach into the clinical setting. The information gathered in the patient interview must be integrated into the medical record. Some settings use formats that are idiosyncratic to their settings. There are a number of formats that have received more widespread acceptance; the HOAC method is one.[21] The format that has received the widest acceptance is the Weed system, or the Problem-Oriented Medical Record (POMR),[22] which will be described in detail. The "SOAP" note is written into the daily patient record. In the SOAP format, S stands for "subjective" and traditionally contains the statement of the patient's presenting complaints. O stands for "objective" findings as a result of observations, tests, and measurements made by the therapist. The A section of the SOAP note contains the therapist's "assessment" or interpretation of the implications of the subjective and objective findings. Last, the P portion represents the "plan" for remediating impairments and disabilities.

The data generated as to concerns can be placed in the S portion of the SOAP. However, rather than merely listing the first or presenting statement, the opportunity exists to list the several concerns and then the major concern, showing the evolution in the exploration step. Alternatively, one may list the major concern after it has been selected and specified in accordance with the procedures described in the previous chapter.

Therapists in clinical practice are concerned with making the entire interview efficient while still maximizing patient participation. It is important to keep in mind that the aim is merely to maximize patient participation. While it is not necessary to remain at a free-choice level, it is necessary to be aware of when one is moving to a lower level of participation. If one finds it necessary to do so, it is with the understanding that any reduction in the level of participation may reduce the degree of patient commitment. Such commitment will be important not only in achieving the goals but also in any later part of the ongoing planning cycle. When integrating patient participation in planning into the clinical record, one would describe the degree of participation by the patient in generating the statements. One would record alongside the data the lowest level of participation required in order to generate that data. For example, in answering the question regarding concerns, if the patient required moving to "forced choice" in the specification step but dealt with the exploration step on a "free choice" level, the final product described in the SOAP note would have documentation of the need for "forced choice." It is ultimately the lowest level of participation that would limit the commitment made.

The data generated as to patient goals can be placed in the P portion of the SOAP note. However, it is essential to maintain the distinction between goals and means. The word *plan* in most clinical settings is understood to describe the activities or actions to be taken. However, it has been useful to use the *plan* section of a SOAP note to describe goals also. We have found it helpful to maintain this distinction between goals and means throughout and have designated the goal as the initial portion of any plan; thus the goals generated with the patient can be designated as "P-1" and can contain both short-term and long-term goals. One could specify the goals of highest priority. Once again there should be some statement describing the degree of patient participation in relation to the goal. It may be recalled that the plan will incorporate patient input at this time not only in the goal but in the time line, which could be designated as "P-2." Patient input into the third aspect, or means, will be discussed in the next chapter and could be designated as the third component of the plan, or "P-3."

Data elicited in the evaluation of outcome has not been dealt with explicitly in the Weed system. When this approach to planning has been used in conjunction with the SOAP note, it has appeared appropriate to therapists in clinical practice to place data regarding outcome at the start of the note in the S portion, because it is "subjective" in origin. One may list all the outcomes generated in the exploration step, or the one outcome that was selected and specified. Along with this information would be a statement of lowest degree of patient participation in the making of this statement. This information must be somehow distinguished from the subsequent data in the S portion of the note dealing with the revised concerns. An example would be: S: Outcomes: Made a grilled cheese sandwich once for lunch on Tuesday last week at home. [Level of patient participation: "multiple choice"] Concerns: Pain in left shoulder going down arm interferes with daily activities. [Level of participation: "Free choice"]

The approach to planning described in this book is dynamic, not static. It can be responsive to changes in the patient from hour to hour or from month to month, depending on the situation. The approach can be implemented on a very formal basis with the use of forms such as those found in the exercises. It can also be used informally in daily therapeutic conversations with the patient, then recorded periodically in whatever medical record system in use in any given facility.

## APPLICATION TO ONESELF

As usual, the reader should start by applying the question to personal issues relative to the goals of this book; that is, the student/clinician acts first to do for oneself what one will later do for the patient. The reader should first perform his or her own evaluation of the outcome of the educational program thus far, before redefining the problems and goals for the continuation of the educational program, including the development of a time line for oneself for reevaluation. It is important to note that the principle is that the student has set goals for herself or himself which may be different from or the same as those which have been set by the instructor in the course. It is those personal goals which are now being evaluated and revised.

In addressing the question of what results have been achieved in relation to your previous goals, the student should follow the pattern already established. One would explore several outcomes before selecting the outcome about which one feels the best or the one that one remembers the best, and then specify that particular outcome. The actual results or achievements should meet 4 criteria of specificity. That is, the statement as to outcome would include *what* was achieved, *where* and *when* it happened, and *to what degree*. As a result of defining outcomes, remaining concerns and appropriate goals for the future will become clearer. The rate of accomplishment may have been greater than expected or less, and so the time line may change. Once concerns have been identified, existing goals may need to be modified in some way or a new goal may need to be created.

One student who successively carried out this cyclical process illustrated the relationship between the original concerns and the goals, the relationship of outcomes to goals, and the establishment of new goals in relation to new concerns. Her major concern during the early portion of her first clinical rotation was "being able to ask appropriate questions during the clinical interview to the extent of getting a specific goal." In order to deal with this concern, she set a goal of "getting a specific goal during my 3 remaining interviews without feeling awkward and without direction."

When reviewing the outcomes, she described herself as "successful in controlling the direction of conversation during the last interview to the extent of getting a specific goal." She then became concerned about the timing of the interview for the first time. "I don't feel sure about when to initiate this goal-planning process with a patient." Her aim for her second clinical rotation was to become clearer as to how to use this goal-setting approach most effectively.

When reviewing her second clinical rotation, this same student described herself as "better able to ask appropriate questions and more comfortable during the interview." Her concern now dealt with integrating this approach so that it was flexible and compatible with herself. Many students move in this same way from more technical concerns to the more abstract concerns such as those this student expressed.

Review the goals you listed for yourself in the exercise in Chapter 2. Now use the format in Table 3–1 to evaluate your results in dealing with those personal professional concerns and goals relative to mastering the approach described in this book. Then list those concerns which remain or have newly arisen. List your goals for the next interim of time and specify at least one of them. You can use this same format to reevaluate your performance in an ongoing way throughout your professional career. Remember that you do not have to use the level of participation line when working on your own personal goals. Be sure the exercise is expressed in personal terms: I am concerned that; I will; and so forth. Try to do the exercise on your own first, then if you need

---

**TABLE 3-1. Program Planning Sheet 2 (PPS-2)**

Name _____ Date _____
Therapist _____

1. **What results have you achieved?** (List at least 3.) Select your best result with asterisk and have that statement meet the 4 criteria of "specificity."




   Lowest level of participation _____

2. **What problems do you have? What questions do you have?** (List at least 3.) Select your greatest concern with an asterisk and have that statement meet the 3 criteria of "specificity."




   Lowest level of participation _____

3. **What would you like to see accomplished that would make you feel that you are making some progress in dealing with your greatest concern?** (List 3 and specify the most important one with 3 criteria.)




   Lowest level of participation _____

---

TABLE 3-2. **Example of Student Use of Form 2, Completed after a Patient Interview, during a Part-Time Clinical Rotation**

1. **What results have you achieved?** (List at least 3.) Select your best result with an asterisk and have that statement meet the criteria of "specificity."
   A. I have learned when open-ended questions, suggestions, recommendations, and prescriptions are appropriate during an interview.
   B. I have learned how to differentiate between a goal and a means during an interview.
   *C. I have learned how to interview a patient following the guidelines learned in my clinical problem-solving class, in clinic, during regular therapy time, to the degree that when I interview patients in the clinic they can generate 3 concerns, a main concern, 3 goals, and a specific goal which is relevant to the main concern.

2. **What problems do you have now? What questions do you have?** (List at least 3.) Select your greatest concern with an asterisk and have that statement meet the criteria of "specificity."
   A. I am concerned that I do not yet have enough medical knowledge to always know whether the goals set by a patient are within reason.
   *B. I would like to learn how to respond to a patient during an interview when he sets a goal that is in all likelihood not attainable, to the degree that I can get him to set a short-term goal that is reasonable.
   C. I would like to learn what to do if, during an interview, none of the goals the patient is concerned with are things that relate to therapy.

3. **What would you like to see accomplished which would make you feel that you are making some progress in dealing with your greatest concern?** (List 3 and specify 1.)
   A. That I am realistic in response to an unobtainable goal
   B. That I not reject a patient's goal if it appears to be unobtainable
   *C. That if a patient states an unobtainable goal, I can redirect him toward making a goal that is obtainable, but still let him make the goal in the clinic where he is receiving therapy to the degree that his goal is within reason based on his medical situation

**Time line:** By the end of this semester

---

**TABLE 3-3. Illustration of the Use of Form 2 by a Student after Several Patient Interviews**

1. **What results have you achieved?** (List at least 3.) Select your best result with an asterisk and have that statement meet the criteria of specificity.
   A. I have developed the ability to elicit important concerns from patients.
   B. I have developed the ability to convert concerns into goals that meet the criteria of specificity.
   *C. I have developed the ability to prioritize goals using the weight-sharing system with patients in occupational therapy practice when I interview them during therapy.

2. **What problems do you have? What questions do you have?** (List at least 3.) Select your greatest concern with an asterisk and have that statement meet the criteria of specificity.
   *A. I have difficulty explaining the weight-sharing system to patients so that they understand the process in a short period of time (less than 2 minutes) in a clinical setting.
   B. What are the results of writing goals this way versus other methods (that is, are patients more motivated for treatment)?
   C. How do I use this method to elicit appropriate goals from patients who are unrealistic in their expectations?

3. **What would you like to see accomplished that would make you feel that you are making some progress in dealing with your greatest concern?** (List 3 and specify 1.)
   *A. I would like to be able to develop 3 specific methods of explaining the weight-sharing system that can be used with patients on my next affiliation.
   B. I would like to be able to redirect patients to develop realistic goals.
   C. I would like to be able to elicit goals from patients and form them to meet the criteria of specificity in a short amount of time.

**Time line:** By the end of my spring affiliation

---

some help or suggestions from others, turn to the examples of what other students have done (Tables 3–2, 3–3). Note that the outstanding achievement in the student's mind has an asterisk in front of it, and it is specified to 4 criteria (what, where, when, and degree). The concern and goal that are selected as primary are specified to 3 criteria (what, where *or* when, degree) as discussed in Chapter 2. Time lines are also specified. In Table 3–2 the rather lengthy goal statement is still somewhat vague in terms of degree, but it is still acceptable. Note the goal statement at the end of Table 3–2; it contains the 3 criteria of specificity but not in the usual order.

## APPLICATION TO PATIENT CARE

The student/therapist helps the patient define the problem and then specify an appropriate goal with the maximal degree of participation, as discussed in Chapter 2. Again, we want to emphasize that this is done with the therapist, who uses scientifically based procedures and provides information to the patient to guide the planning process. It is the responsibility of the therapist to do this in order to practice ethically and to meet legal requirements.

Table 3–1 is Program Planning Sheet 2 (PPS–2), which may now be used by the reader as an exercise. Please copy this form and use it to interview the people and patients whom you have previously interviewed. This form contains a place for defining the level of participation required in order to meet the objectives of the interview in answering each of the questions. For example, a patient working with a student therapist using PPS–1 described her concerns as follows: (1) I can't lift my right arm; (2) I can't comb my hair with my right arm; and (3) I can't wash windows in my apartment. When asked to select, she identified her major concern as "I can't comb my hair," and she confirmed her selection. In setting a goal for her therapy, she eventually specified her goal to be "I would like to be able to comb my hair with my right hand here in the hospital without any pain in my shoulder." In setting this goal, her lowest level of participation was at the multiple choice level.

Evaluation may occur at any time—hourly, daily, weekly, monthly—depending on the patient's condition and, to some extent, the type of facility, regulations from third-party payers, and similar realities. The first step in the review process consists of identifying any outcomes achieved, particularly in relation to the goal(s) initially set, but not limited to that. Statements of outcome are most useful when they are specified (what, where, when, and to what degree) with maximum patient participation. In the case cited above, the student therapist using PPS–2 reviewed the patient's plan and progress with the patient after 2 weeks. The outcomes in this instance were as follows: (1) I can comb my hair without pain in my right shoulder; (2) I can reach things in my kitchen cabinets without any right-arm pain; and (3) I can drive my car without pain such as when I go to the store near my house. The lowest level of patient participation in making these statements was at the multiple choice level.

In light of the outcomes listed in the paragraph above, this patient, guided by her therapist, listed the following residual concerns: (1) The back of my shoulder feels tight; (2) I can't move my right arm very fast when I hold it over my head; and (3) I have some soreness between my shoulder and my spine. She selected and confirmed the second statement as her greatest concern. The goal for the future she specified to be "To move my right arm as fast as I need when it is over my head, without pain."

**TABLE 3–4. Patient's Medical Record Using a Narrative System and Incorporating the Contents of PPS–1.**

**HPI:** A 56-year-old white female referred for evaluation and treatment by Dr. S. Her chief complaint is pain and stiffness in the right shoulder, especially when doing activities which involve using the RUE above the head. The symptoms have not changed significantly over the last month and began insidiously approximately 4 months ago. The pain is described as an ache which is increased with overhead activities (e.g., combing hair, reaching into cabinets, etc.) and relieved with rest. Patient denies a PMH of a similar problem.

**Problem Statements:** Patient is concerned that (1) *pain prevents her from combing her hair when it needs it, so that it looks good; (2) she cannot reach into overhead cabinets in her kitchen without discomfort; and (3) she has to ask her husband to help her with housework. Patient was cooperative; concerns were elicited with open-ended questions.

**Goals:** Patient will be able to comb and arrange her hair to her satisfaction, whenever needed, without pain by the end of 2 weeks. Goals were listed using multiple-choice questions.

**Evaluation:**
*Neck:* negative during upper quarter scan (AROM, PROM, accessory motion tests, special tests, and palpation).
*AROM R shoulder:* abduction 0–100°, flexion 0–120°, external rotation 35°, internal rotation 55°. Patient reports a 4 level pain at end-range flexion and rotations. L shoulder WNL without pain.
*PROM R shoulder:* abduction 0–110°, flexion 0–130°, external rotation 35°, internal rotation 60°. The chief complaint is reproduced during all motions with end-range PROM. End feel is capsular with flexion, internal rotation, and abduction; external rotation produces a spasm end feel.
*Resistive isometric tests:* decreased ability to generate tension with abduction, producing pain; all other motions are WNL without pain.
*Accessory motion tests:* anterior and inferior glide are decreased compared with uninvolved side; all others are WNL; all are without pain.
*Palpation:* unable to reproduce CC with palpation locally and from all dermatomally related structures.
*Posture:* no significant postural deviations.

**Working hypothesis:** Patient is unable to comb hair and reach into cabinets without pain because of inflammation in the area of the supraspinatus tendon, decreased AROM (flexion and external rotation), and decreased anterior and inferior glide of the humerus.

**Criteria for testing the hypothesis:** No pain with resisted abduction; AROM flexion to 150° and external rotation to 60° without pain; anterior and inferior glide of the humerus equal to uninvolved side.

**Treatment strategy:**

**Treatment specifics:**

## TABLE 3-5. The Concerns and Goals Portion of a SOAP Note

**HPI and PMH**
1/14/87. 38-year-old white female referred for evaluation and treatment of an acute (R) knee strain which happened 1/10/87 while the patient was playing tennis. Patient reports hearing a "pop" in the (R) knee after (R) ankle plantarflexed and inverted. Following these events, patient reports falling down. No trauma to ankle. PMH unremarkable.

**S:**
Patient is worried about
    1. not being able to drive,
    2. falling down and injuring the knee more severely, and
  *3. not being able to play tennis.

**P:**
Patient Goals
    1. Wants knee to be "normal like the way it was before my injury" while she is playing a singles and a doubles
        to the degree that she can play without pain in the knee.
    2. Wants to be able to participate in physical activities with family members in her free time
        without pain in the (R) knee.
  *3. Wants to be able to exercise independently in her free time
        without pain in the (R) knee.
Concerns were elicited with open-ended questions; goals required multiple-choice options on 2 occasions.

---

## TABLE 3-6. Narrative, Problem-Solving Format for Recording of Concerns and Goals

1. Initial Data
    2/4/86. 17-year-old male referred from ER by Dr. Dementia for evaluation and treatment of acute (L) ankle sprain which happened this AM during football practice. X-rays negative, patient to take aspirin QID. PMH unremarkable.
    Patient states he hurt his ankle while being tackled during football practice this morning.

2. Problem Statement and Goals
    Patient is worried about (1) being cut from the team, (2) his leg hurts, and (3) (cc) he can't walk on his LLE. These were elicited by giving multiple-choice options on 1 occasion.
    STG: patient will return to normal activity during sporting events (e.g., running, football) and be pain free.
        LTG: 1. full active and passive ROM in therapy, pain free
            2. weight bearing on LLE when walking, pain free
    Patient verbalized these goals in response to open-ended questions.

---

TABLE 3–7. **Example of a Progressive SOAP Note with Regard to System of This Manual, Other Content is Omitted (see Table 2–6)**

---

7-1-87. Initial evaluation
**S:** (elicited with open-ended questions)
   1. Patient cannot play golf once a week with his friends as he did a year ago because holding a golf club in his hand is painful.
   2. Patient cannot spread mayonnaise on bread, open a jar or milk carton when he wants to eat without someone helping him hold the food items.
  *3. Patient cannot dress himself without help from his wife.

   * = Chief complaint

**P:** Goals; elicited with open-ended questions
   1. Patient wants to be able to put on his socks by himself.
   2. Patient wants to put on his pants by himself.
  *3. Patient wants to be able to put on his shirt without help.

   * = Most important goal

7-8-87. Reevaluation
**S:** Results achieved in relation to previous goals; obtained through open-ended questions
   1. Patient can put on shirt by himself in 5–7 minutes.
   2. Patient can tie shoes in less than 10 minutes when getting dressed.
   3. Patient can button and zip trousers.

   New problems: obtained through multiple-choice questions
   1. Patient cannot hold or swing golf club well enough on the golf course to play 1 hole of golf.
   2. Patient does not have enough flexibility to reach down and hold trousers while putting his legs in.
  *3. Patient cannot get his hand behind his back when getting dressed to get belt through the belt loops.

   * = Chief complaint

**P:** Goals; obtained by making recommendations
  *1. Get hand in back when getting dressed so he can get belt through belt loop
   2. Be able to grasp golf club firmly enough on the golf course so he can practice putting, using his L arm to help guide the club
   3. Be able to put his pants on unassisted

**Time line:** To be accomplished in 6 months

These data may be incorporated into a SOAP note or other appropriate medical record. Table 3–4 illustrates the presentation of the above case in the medical record using a more narrative system.[21] There are some differences because the two interviews were done on different days, which illustrates how patient concerns may vary from day to day. Note how the concerns of the authors are woven into the examples in this text, even the asterisk, without disrupting the flow of the narrative. This table uses PPS–1. The goal statement could be considered a short-term goal, and only one is stated; it was selected out of several goals based on concerns. At this point in therapy, the therapist and patient have not yet dealt with the issue of outcomes. This statement also includes a time line.

Tables 3–5 through 3–7 are examples of student interviews of patients written for incorporation into the medical record. Table 3–5 is the simplest form of a SOAP note and provides data relevant to Chapter 2, that is, an initial note containing early concerns and goals. Note that there is a sequence in these 3 goals, with the first being the most difficult and the third the least difficult. Sometimes one can build sequencing into goal statements by making the hardest goal(s) a long-term one and the least difficult goals short-term ones. In this instance the patient started with the most difficult, but by continuing the exploration step, she began to set successively shorter-term goals. The therapist helped by asking what would be the steps toward accomplishing her overall goal. This illustrates the value of exploration. Table 3–6 is a short but complete narrative note.

Table 3–7 is the most complete example, and it deals with the same patient as in Table 2–6, with evaluation as to outcomes in relation to the initial goal. Note the progression of the patient and the subsequent change in concerns and goals.

# 4

# *Patient as Designer*

## WHAT ARE THE GOALS?

The previous chapters described ways for improving patient participation in therapy by enabling the patient to take as active a role as possible in setting goals, evaluating the outcomes, and making revised goals in the light of the changing character of the patient's concerns.

Thus far we have not discussed the participation of the patient in the definition of the treatment program or the means by which the goals are to be achieved. It has been assumed that the treatment program, at least initially, had been recommended by the therapist who then sought the patient's agreement to the program to be followed. A *plan* consists not only of goals and a time line for the evaluation of outcomes but the means to be used to achieve the goals. The participation of the patient in the ongoing evaluation and revision process provides an opportunity to participate in answering this important component of a plan in collaboration with the therapist. One aim of this chapter is to enable the student/clinician to specify the means (treatment procedures/equipment) with maximal patient participation as part of an ongoing relatonship. Another goal of this chapter is to illustrate even further the integration of this approach into the clinical setting.

# WHAT ARE THE PROBLEMS?

## EVALUATING EFFICACY

Failure in carrying out the recommended actions is what is generally described as "noncompliance." The lack of follow-through by patients contributes to making the evaluation of the outcomes in health care so difficult. In order to determine the efficacy of the procedures one needs to evaluate not only the outcomes but the relationship of any outcomes to the antecedent activities. For an activity to be "efficacious," it must be viewed as having the power to produce a desired effect. Not only must there be the desired effect, but a relationship must be established between the action(s) taken and the outcomes of those actions.

The additional question as to means can be asked after having described some of the outcomes achieved. This fourth question to be used in planning with the patient is *what may have helped to bring about the results?* Evocation of the scene in terms of where and when the outcomes were achieved can provide the context for defining the actions taken that were helpful. One is thus seeking to determine the efficacy of the procedures recommended initially.

In addition, the data so generated can be incorporated into the plan for the future. The actions that were helpful can be carried on further with confirmation on the part of the patient and therapist that they were actually useful in this particular instance. At the very least, such ongoing use of successful methods can be seen to be relevant to the continued management of the same sort of problem as the one initially stated. The methods successful in the past may, however, even contribute to the solution of what may be seen as a new problem. Student/therapists have difficulty seeing how one may use methods that worked in one situation to help achieve future goals dealing with new problems. It is important to recognize that there may be more ability to generalize the use of methods than might at first be apparent.

The exploration of at least 3 actions or 3 aspects of any 1 action is designed to increase the awareness on the part of the patient that options do exist, as well as an awareness of what those options are. In many instances a person becomes a patient and enters therapy after having lost some of the ways by which he or she ordinarily performs activities significant to everyday life. An important part of the rehabilitative process is recognition of alternative ways of doing things, of adapting or compensating. These ways are by definition "abnormal" in that they are usually different from the ways the person has accomplished these same everyday goals in the past. They may also be different from the ways most people carry out those activities. It is important in the interaction between therapist and patient that there be use of every possible opportunity to increase the sense that there is more than 1 way to do something. If there are only 2 ways, there is still a sense of limited choice. Describing 3 answers to the question as to *what worked?* opens up even more the sense of freedom, of options.

In the exploration step of answering this question, as with the other questions used thus far, it is essential that the answers arise to the maximal extent possible from the patient. One may start with open-ended questions and move to lower degrees of participation, as needed, to elicit the several different answers.

The subsequent selection step can be based once again upon any of the techniques used up to now. The basis for making the decision as to one's choice may relate to the actions that seemed to work the best or that are the clearest in one's mind. Another basis for selection can relate to the important issue of the source of the actions that were helpful. Emphasis would be on those actions carried out mainly by the client or the particular contribution that the person with the disability made to the actions that were effective. In working with persons with disabilities one can strengthen the entire process of rehabilitation by recognition of the contribution of the patient to the outcomes achieved.

A major effect of impairment has been the sense of loss of control of one's body with serious implications for a sense of loss of control in one's life. The development of a sense of personal contribution to the achievement of positive outcomes can be a crucial component of the ultimate goal of regaining a sense of control over one's destiny. The sense that the actions leading to success have been taken by the patient rather than some outside agent is an important aspect of the development of a sense of efficacy of the person involved. It is personal efficacy in problem solving that is a goal, along with a greater degree of awareness of some of the ways such outcomes were achieved. The basis for selection might be *Which of these actions did you contribute to the most?* or *What did you do to help?*

During the exploration step, if the patient states only 1 idea of what may have helped, then further exploration may be focused on what actions the person may have contributed. One example is when "hot packs" was the one answer to the question as to what may have helped. In dealing with the further exploration as to what the client may have contributed to the effect of the hot pack, one can offer suggestions such as "heating the hot packs," "putting them on the prescribed place," "making sure they stay on for the whole time." Even if medication was the only choice, it is possible to ascribe the effects at least in part to the acts of the patient in taking the medication, in the proper dosage and at the proper time intervals.

If several ideas as to what worked arise during the exploration step, then the selection may be based upon the action to which the patient may have contributed the most. For example, one person ascribed the improvement in his spasms to "warmer weather," "stretching exercise," and use of a specific medication. During the selection step, he chose the stretching exercises when the basis for selection was the action to which he contributed the most.

The specification of the selected actions should describe *what* actions were taken to a greater degree of specificity than used in the examples thus far. A higher degree of specificity is appropriate when addressing the technical characteristics of either equipment or treatment programs. An exercise program, for example, should be described in terms such as "swim 30 minutes in the pool at the health club every other day at a peak pulse rate of 130/minute.' Such a statement specifies not only what is to be done and where but also how long, how often, and how fast. The actions to be taken generally require a greater degree of specification than has been used up to now in reference to the problem statement or the goal statement. Five points of specificity are thus sought, with particular emphasis on describing not only *how long* but also *how much*. For example, a treatment program could be described as "apply hot packs (130°F) to the left shoulder 3 times daily for 30 minutes each time" that would meet the 5 points for specificity. Still another example would be "apply the postoperative arthroplasty splint each day for 22 hours a day to the extensor surface for the next 2 weeks." This statement includes *what* was done, *where*, *when*, *how long*, and *how often*.

## REVISION OF TREATMENT PROGRAMS

The use of this question as to "means" involves the patient as a designer just as previously we have dealt with the patient as a planner and as an evaluator. The problem of noncompliance has been discussed earlier with the suggestion that the setting of more relevant goals would be helpful. Failure to take medication, to follow through with a treatment program, or to use the equipment designed to help can also arise from the lack of "fit" of the actions to be carried out. The timing of the treatments, their frequency, or their complexity can make it more or less likely that the program will be followed. The equipment may be too small, too large, or in some other way inappropriate.

If the review process explores what may have helped in a nonjudgmental way, the opportunity exists for the client to participate in increasing the "fit" of the procedures by providing information as to what specific aspects of the actions originally recommended were carried out. If the interaction permits the patient a wide latitude for making free contributions, there is a greater likelihood that the patient will describe modifications of the original recommendations that the person made on his or her own. For example, although the original recommendation may have been to apply a splint for an hour several times each day but the patient reports that he actually applied it once a day, the new *plan* for the future can now include recognition of the procedures or means that were actually effective.

Occasionally, the patient will describe some new idea that seemed to work. One example is that of a man with spasms that interfered with his ability to push his wheelchair and go outdoors. He reported some improvement which he attributed to the stretching exercises that had been recommended. When asked as to what else may have helped, he also mentioned that he had started using ice in the area of pain. He would apply it soon after he began to feel pain in his back after sitting up for long periods. The use of ice became part of his program. The plan for the future could thus include patient contributions not only to the goal and time line but to the means or programs as well. Those ideas which arose from the patient's own experimentation or were actions he or she describes as actually carrying out are far more likely to be carried out again rather than actions attributed to some outside agent not generally under the control of the patient. Moreover, attentive listening to the patient by the therapist can lead to an increase in the options that can be offered to subsequent patients. The entire process of addressing the question of means can thus validate the patient's own problem-solving ideas and can lead to his or her being an even more active participant in his or her own care.

Enabling the client/patient to participate in the design of his or her therapy offers the greatest opportunity for increasing the effectiveness of the entire interaction between the professional therapist and the person with disabilities. The degree of participation could be expected to increase in the process of an ongoing relationship with a person with disabilities. Particularly in the design of equipment, the opportunity exists for the person with disabilities to become increasingly knowledgeable of modes for the adaptation of technical aids, such as wheelchairs, to his or her own needs. With increasing contribution of the person with disabilities to the design of one's own treatment programs, therapists can grow in their own skills by having additional ideas to offer to subsequent patients. The patients are thus enlisted to help solve not only their own problems but also problems faced by others.[23]

The following example drawn from the design of an appropriate wheelchair can illustrate the application of the principles being described. This 35-year-old man had a recent injury to his spinal cord with a neurologic level at C-6. During the early postinjury phase, the user described a number of goals or criteria for evaluation of a wheelchair that would fit his needs. One goal was to be able to balance himself while sitting so that he would still be able to use both his arms in carrying out tasks without needing to hook one arm over the back of the chair to balance himself. Another concern he felt was important was to be able to remove his armrests easily in light of his lack of finger dexterity. Still another personal goal dealt with his plans to travel widely as he had prior to his injury. He therefore wanted a wheelchair that could be easily taken apart and stored in a relatively small space. Another high priority for this person, who also happened to be diabetic, was to be able to maintain his physical health and cardiovascular endurance.

In selecting the means for meeting these goals, the patient had the opportunity, on his request, to use a lightweight wheelchair with a variety of levels of back support. He learned that he could counterbalance his weight by leaning rather far back and thus have both arms free to carry out other tasks. When he had been fitted to a chair with a high back more consistent with the usual method for dealing with problems in balance, he had been unable to use the weight of his trunk to counterbalance and so needed to use one of his arms to steady himself. Thus he was able to contribute, on the basis of his own experience, the value of a back support lower than ordinarily recommended. In this instance, as in others in which design issues arise, the principle is not just the particular back height but other design factors as well, which may vary depending on the individual user and his or her characteristics and priorities.

The selection of what might be other appropriate means for meeting his several goals was aided by a magazine article in which there had been a listing of the several alternatives now available in lightweight wheelchairs. "I knew what the options were myself. I had a chance to think things through for myself before finally selecting the parts I needed." These options included a freely movable rotating armrest as well as a chair that could be modified to use for exercise and to be easily broken down to be stored.

At the time of review some months after discharge, this patient described his wheelchair as meeting his needs well. He had been able to take several airplane trips; balance was not a problem; and he had been able to participate in wheelchair slalom racing regularly. An initial concern of the staff that his lightweight chair would interfere with his ability to carry out transfers without a transfer board had not turned out to be a problem.

The issue is not the particular components that this person helped select. No single wheelchair is appropriate for everyone, even given the same level of injury. What is significant is the methodology by which the appropriate wheelchair components can be selected, with particular emphasis on the degree of user participation permitted. This user functioned at the level of "free choice" in respect to setting goals and at the level of "multiple choice" in selecting the means for meeting those goals by having available to him the options to review. This user probably also functioned at a much higher level of participation than most are able to achieve. The principle is that he was given the maximal opportunity to participate rather than the level of participation that was actually achieved. One may find far more contributions to be made and more effective use of technology and treatments that incorporate such contributions.

## INTEGRATION INTO THE CLINICAL SETTING

In narrative notes, the answers to the question as to "What worked?" can now be incorporated as part of the total plan for the next interim. One may recall that the term *plan* consists of a goal, means, and a time line. The means by which the goal is to be achieved is the new component, which can now reflect the contribution of the patient to the ideas as to what worked. It is particularly clear if the identified problem is ongoing that the activities that have worked may be continued with additional confirmation of their validity. There are illustrations of the use of such information in the exercises in the last part of this chapter.

The integration into the clinical record of this new question as to what worked can go on while using the format of the SOAP note. The place in the SOAP format for incorporating this new information can be in the S portion where the outcomes have been placed and would appropriately follow the data as to outcomes and precede the data as to new concerns. The lowest level of participation required in order to elicit the answer should be described. Once such data have been generated in collaboration with the patient, they can be used to complete the *plan* by filling in the means in the P portion of the SOAP note. The means already deemed somewhat effective can now be integrated into the plan for future outcomes. The client can now contribute the means in addition to the goal and time line to formulate all aspects of a total plan.

Still another method of integrating this approach into the clinical setting is to recognize how one may vary the questions addressed in any one situation. It is not always necessary to use the entire set of questions as illustrated up to now. It is helpful merely to recognize that there is an appropriate pairing of questions: One can ask about goals in relation to concerns; about outcomes in relation to previous goals; about what may have helped in relation to outcomes. One may choose to ask only one question at any particular session. For example, once overall goals have been established, it could be appropriate to explore outcomes in relation to those initial goals at the end of each therapy session rather than await the total completion of the plan. During the session itself, it may be useful to explore with the patient what may have worked right at the time when he or she managed to accomplish even a portion of the total outcome sought. For example, when a man with hemiplegia was able to walk even a short distance, he was asked about what had worked. He then described what he had done that had been helpful to accomplish that feat. His description helped him continue to carry out that action in the next attempt at walking.

Eliciting answers to the question as to what actions may have helped is particularly valuable as an integral part of the therapeutic setting. The description of the actions that were taken may be very simple. It is particularly important that they be described in terms that reflect instructions that the patient can give himself or herself. Those instructions are brought to a conscious level in interaction with the therapist. The therapist gives evidence, by feedback, of having heard the person make the statement. In the context of having evidence of being heard lies a greater opportunity for the person to hear the instruction for himself or herself. By hearing oneself say the instruction, one then will be more likely to later instruct oneself on one's own. Eventually these instructions can be internalized.

When offering ideas in the multiple-choice format, the therapist should describe actions in terms of relatively simple instructions, such as in the example that follows. The man with hemiplegia who stood between 2 parallel bars for the first time was asked immediately after having done so what he did that may have helped that happen. When he could not respond on a "free choice" level, he was offered several suggestions. He chose "locking my knee." He also chose the idea offered of "holding on with my arms." When asked as to any other ideas, he mentioned freely on his own "knowing what I was trying to do." All these actions could be used again in continuing to strive to improve his walking. In addition, the last statement, one that he made on his own, dealt with the general principle of setting goals. This was an action that could apply to a far larger number of situations than merely one of walking, although the idea came to the patient's awareness in the context of solving this particular problem.

## APPLICATION TO ONESELF

As in the previous chapters, the therapist can best learn how to work with this new question as to the actions that helped by applying the question to oneself prior to doing so with the client. Use the form found in Table 4–1 for this purpose.

In exploring the question as to means, it is important to list at least 3 aspects before selecting which one may have made the greatest contribution. Then specify it to meet the 5-point criteria. The other aspect to keep in mind is that the answers to the question as to what worked which arise in the context of the outcomes already achieved can now be used as part of the plan for the future, in which you consider *how* to accomplish new goals.

With the use of the format found in Table 4–1, several therapists in training evaluated their performances in carrying out several interviews with patients. The selected outcome of one student included "learning during the interview that my patient was more insightful than I thought." In reference to that outcome, the student/therapist explored this new question as to what may have helped bring about that result. The following answers arose out of the use of the question *What worked?* "giving the patient control," "using the format of the structured interview process," and "focusing on patient activities rather than on pain." When the student was asked to select which activity was most under her control, she selected "using the format of the structured interview process." She went on further to say, "I knew what I was doing." The emphasis in this exercise is on what you, the student/therapist, did that helped bring about the outcome you achieved. Later, when the question regarding what worked is applied to patients, the emphasis will be on what the patient did to bring about the results achieved.

A therapist in an in-service training program described her achievements in the application of this method as follows: "Patients will generally set their own goals; I can get more of a measurable achievement; I'm more aware of doing things in a more logical, quantitative way. What outcome was most

important to me was: I wasn't stuck as much in a rut. I'm trying new things."
In answer to the question as to what may have helped, she reported, "I discussed the new methods with my classmates, I practiced the techniques with several people before trying it on patients, I kept an open mind, and I watched the instructor work with patients." When asked, "What did *you* do to help?" she answered, "I practiced on my own." Here again, the answers to the questions are in relation to *your* actions. Personalizing the answers concerning your own actions can help you enable patients to do the same.

Tables 4–2, 4–3, and 4–4 illustrate the application of all 5 questions posed in the Introduction to the work in this course by student therapists. Note the relationships among the various parts of these examples; each section flows from (i.e., is related to) the previous one. Note particularly that in Tables 4–2 and 4–3 the means written into the *plan* are based on "What worked" in question 2.

A word needs to be said about flexibility. A student/therapist reported the success with which she was able to integrate the various questions of the planning process into her day-to-day work with her patients during her summer rotation. She found that her patients accepted very readily her asking them the question regarding concerns. She would ask it "straight out." Her clients would tell her about their problems, and she could then focus them and help them be specific about goals.

She would use questions in a conversational way. While she was ranging the patient's limbs, she would ask what he or she felt was being accomplished. She found that the patients became more enthusiastic and carried that enthusiasm over into other aspects of their lives in the hospital. She felt that what helped bring about the participation she was getting was that the patients knew that someone was listening. Using the question "Why do you want to come to therapy?" was a way to get across the idea of setting goals. The patient comes with a purpose and more and more tells the therapist what he needs to get done in any particular session. He sets more reasonable goals and takes it one step at a time. She felt what worked was: asking questions rather than giving orders, giving the patients time to talk, acting as though the patient is a real partner in therapy, and being specific about the goals.

## APPLICATION TO PATIENT CARE

You are now ready to lead a patient through the entire cycle of planning using all 5 questions about concerns, goals, outcomes, what worked, and a total plan. And you should be able to do this with as much patient participation in the process as possible.

Copy Table 4–1 and use it to interview several people: peers, family, patients. Try it yourself first, then look at the example we have provided in Table 4–5. Table 4–5 illustrates the full process that has been discussed in this

---

**TABLE 4-1.  Program Planning Sheet 3 (PPS-3)**

Name _____  Date _____
                                        Therapist _____

1. **What results have you achieved?** (List at least 3.) Select your best result with asterisk and have that statement meet the criteria of "specificity."




   Level of participation _____

2. **What actions did you take that may have helped to bring about those results?** (List at least 3.) Select what you feel was most helpful and meet the criteria of "specificity" for that statement using an asterisk.




   Level of participation _____

3. **What problems do you have now? What questions do you have?** (List at least 3.) Select your greatest concern with an asterisk and have that statement meet the criteria of "specificity."




   Level of participation _____

4. **What would you like to see accomplished that would make you feel that you are making some progress in dealing with your greatest concern?** (List 3.)




   Level of participation _____

5. **What is your plan?**
   A. **GOAL** (Please be specific)
      What?
      Setting?
      To what degree?
   B. **MEANS** (Identify from those actions which may have worked in 2 above)
   C. **Time line**

   Level of participation _____

text. Note how each question and the answer to each question lead into the next question and its answer. Examine your own interview records. Do they flow logically from one question and answer to the next?

Table 4–6 illustrates how the entire process can be documented in the medical record using the Weed system of SOAP notes.[22] Note that any information that comes from the patient's evaluation of the situation is under S, subjective information; this includes concerns, patient's impressions of outcomes, and what worked. If the therapist has other impressions about concerns, outcomes, or efficacy of treatment, and/or if the information is based on measured data, it should go under O, observations. It should go under A, assessment, if it is a professional judgment. Goals and plans go under P, plan, separated, if necessary, into patient goals and therapist goals. For example, in this table goals 4 and 5 are therapist goals and reflect a more kinesiologic orientation. Both S and P should contain statements of level of patient participation in arriving at the information recorded there. Also note that under "what worked" each of the three items relates to a different outcome in the section above it; and under "P₁: Goals" the first three goals relate to each of the three concerns listed above. This is a perfectly acceptable alternative to having "what worked" and "goals" relate only to the most important outcomes or concerns. Note also the flexible use of the format, for example, 8 goals instead of 3.

The following is an example of the application to patient care of the question as to what worked. It also illustrates the application of several of the other questions, all within a 15-minute session in a flexible format.

> I was assigned to work with an elderly man who was lying in bed with restraints on both wrists and his side rails up. He was lying flat on his back and opened his eyes when I came in. His speech was slurred and somewhat hoarse. He seemed to be emotionally labile and would start to cry as he spoke in answer to my questions. I knew that he had been seen by a previous therapist but his confusion was too great for her to work with him earlier in the week. When I asked him what was troubling him, he first pointed to his restraints and tried to pull them off. I asked him if he wanted them off and he nodded "yes." I took them off and followed with a

---

**TABLE 4-2. Example of Student Use, at the End of a Week of Full-Time Clinical Study, of PPS-3 Concerning Her Own Interests**

---

1. What results have you achieved?
   A. I have been more successful in terms of controlling the direction of conversation during the patient interview for the duration of the interview.
   B. I feel that I am now able to document and understand patient's concerns/goals while conducting the interview so that I can gather appropriate information related to the patient's problem.
  *C. I was able to work with the patient ( we were a team)
       during an interview
       at the hospital
       in the time allotted (20 minutes).

2. What actions/means were used to produce those results?
   A. I had several opportunities to observe a therapist demonstrate relevant skills while working with patients.
  *B. It was helpful that I was responsible for developing SOAP notes
       (goal statements)
       in the clinic
       during my rotation
       for at least one patient each day
       on my own.
   C. It was helpful to interact with patient and therapists daily for a week.

3. What problems do you still have?
  *A. I still have some trouble thinking of appropriate questions to ask
       during the interview
       so that I feel comfortable during the interview.
   B. I don't know enough about therapy at this point.
   C. I feel inexperienced talking to patients.

4. What are your goals?
   A. talk more with patients
   B. study therapy methods
  *C. conduct an interview using questions
       during my next clinical experience
       to the degree that both patient and I feel that we have set
         meaningful goals for therapy

5. What is your plan?
   Goal: Conduct several interviews with a patient in clinic and
         generate a goal acceptable to both patient and me without
         feeling uncomfortable during the interview
   Means: Practice by being responsible for writing SOAP notes
          watch others interview patients
          get feedback from others when I interview
   Time line: By the end of my next full-time clinical experience

---

**TABLE 4-3. Example of Student Use of Form PPS-3**

---

1. What results have you achieved?
   *A. Able to ask more appropriate, direct questions
       during interview
       in clinic
       so that PPS-3 was completed in 20 minutes
    B. able to manage time allotted
    C. able to encourage patient without leading him

2. What actions helped to bring about those results?
   *A. I practiced the process
       with family and friends
       as often as possible
       after class
       to the degree that I had the form memorized
    B. read patient's history before interview
    C. reviewed previous interviews and studied my mistakes

3. What problems remain?
    A. still feel uncomfortable interviewing patients
    B. have problems isolating a specific goal
   *C. dealing with a variety of patient concerns
       in clinical settings
       so that I feel comfortable

4. What would you like to see yourself accomplishing in the future
   which would make you feel that you were making progress in
   dealing with your concerns?
    A. I would like to be able to complete an initial interview in 15
       minutes or less.
   *B. I would like to interview several patients with different
          problems
       in clinic
       and feel comfortable no matter what the problem.
    C. I would like to be able to isolate one specific goal and specify
       it.

5. What is your plan?
   Goal: Interview any patient
         in a hospital or clinical setting
         and generate a specific goal in fifteen minutes or
         less with maximum patient participation.
   Means: practice interviewing
          as often as possible
          with anyone who is willing
          wherever possible
          and completing each interview within 20 minutes.

   By when: by the end of summer affiliation

TABLE 4-4. **Example of Student Assessment of His Own Educational Plans Relative to Program Planning with Patients**

1. What results have you achieved?
   *A. I understand the importance of using open-ended questions during the interview, in a clinical setting, to the extent that I can achieve more patient participation.
   B. I gained more practical experience in the interview process to the extent that I feel more comfortable.
   C. I have gained more confidence in my ability to conduct an interview with a patient in clinic so that I feel comfortable.

2. What actions helped bring about these results?
   A. listening to interviews done by other therapists
   *B. practicing interviewing with several patients, in clinic, during earlier clinical affiliations, as often as possible.
   C. practicing with students, friends, and family, in class, at home, on weekends, as often as possible

3. What problems remain?
   A. I still feel inexperienced.
   *B. Can I really help patients establish functional goals, during an interview, in clinic, to the degree that they are realistic and specific?
   C. Can I deal effectively with uncooperative patients?

4. What would you like to see happen?
   A. do interviews that result in meaningful goal writing
   B. successfully interview other health professionals
   *C. perform several interviews with patients
   in a clinical setting
   so that the total plan is written to the satisfaction of both the patient and myself

5. What is your plan?
   Goal: Complete several patient *plans*
   in clinic
   so that both of us are satisfied
   Means: practice, practice, practice with different patients every day during the therapy sessions
   By when: the end of the summer clinicals

Name _____   Date _____8-4-88_____
                                        Therapist _____

1. **What results have you achieved?** (List at least 3.) Select your best result with asterisk and have that statement meet the criteria of "specificity."
   A. walk better
   *B. get on and off the bed pan in hospital as needed
   C. turn over better in bed
   Level of participation _____open-ended questions_____

2. **What actions did you take that may have helped to bring about those results?** (List at least 3.) Select what you feel was most helpful and meet the criteria of "specificity" for that statement using an asterisk.
   *A. practiced use of bedpan
       in my room
       each day
       twice a day
       as long as needed
   B. pulling theraband
   C. exercises in bed
   Level of participation _____multiple choice_____

3. **What problems do you have now? What questions do you have?** (List at least 3.) Select your greatest concern with an asterisk and have that statement meet the criteria of "specificity."
   A. want to get up and go home
   *B. need to fix food at home by myself when I get hungry
   C. can't get things ready for cooking at home
   D. can't clean up in kitchen at home after cooking
   Level of participation _____open-ended questions_____

4. **What would you like to see accomplished which would make you feel that you are making some progress in dealing with your greatest concern?** (List 3.)
   A. to be able to get food together and put it away
   *B. to be able to fix a simple meal for myself at home when hungry
   C. be able to wash dishes
   Level of participation _____multiple choice_____

5. **What is your plan?**
   A. **GOAL:** (Please be specific)
       What?          Fix a piece of toast
       Setting?       at home
       To what degree?  without burning myself
   B. **MEANS:** (Identify from those actions which may have worked in 2 above)
       exercises in bed to strengthen my arms and hands, using Theraband, 15-20 minutes a day to the extent that I can depress the toaster button.
       training in O.T. in kitchen skills
   C. **TIME LINE:** by the end of this month
   Level of participation _____multiple choice_____

---

TABLE 4–6.  **Portions of a SOAP Note Illustrating the Incorporation of Data Collected in a PPS–3 Format**

---

**Problems:** (in the POMR chart, these are found on a separate page)
1. L-3 incomplete paraplegia
2. Burst fx s/p CRIF with bone graft @ L-2 to L-4
3. R scapular fx
4. R 5th metatarsal fx
5. Fx of L pubic ramus
   achieved using open-ended questions

**S:** Outcomes:
 *1. I can sit in my wheelchair with less pain in my LLE.
  2. I can bring myself to sitting at bedside with minimal assistance.
  3. I can put my brace on by myself.
What worked:
 *1. By closing my eyes and slowing down my breathing for 5 minutes or less, wherever I am, whenever I have pain in my LLE, I can relieve the sharp pain in my LLE.
  2. By pulling my LEs up to my chest with my UEs, as far as I can without pain, and by sitting up, I can push myself to the side of the bed.
  3. I put the arm rail at the side of the bed to assist me in rolling so that I can put on my brace.
Concerns:
 *1. my hamstrings are too tight to allow me to sit at 90° hip flexion.
  2. I can't reach my LE with one hand and hold myself in sitting with the other hand without assistance.
  3. I can't get my pants on around my ankles without assistance.
Subjective data obtained through multiple-choice questions

**O:** Patient performed transfers w/c < > bed with safety guarding. Patient performed pushups while prone, 10×. Patient is able to come from prone to long sitting with hips flexed at 80°.

**A:** Patient progressing quite well with treatment. Patient seems to be experiencing much less discomfort during sitting. Patient's rehab. activities are restricted by tight hamstrings. Patient is quite motivated for treatment.

$P_1$: (goals)
 *1. to achieve greater ease in performing bed mobility activities and transfers, to the degree that he can come to 90° of hip flexion
  2. Patient wants to be able to bring LEs to the side of the bed independently.
  3. Patient wants to put on pants independently.
  4. increase hamstring flexibility
  5. increase LE strength
  6. independent in bed mobility
  7. independent in long sitting and bench sitting
  8. independent in w/c on uneven surfaces

$P_2$: (means)
Continue present treatment, i.e., slow breathing with eyes closed, pulling LEs to chest, pushing to side of bed, practice putting on brace. Begin sitting balance activities, bed mobility activities, and w/c activities on uneven surfaces.

$P_3$ Time-line: by December 1
Plans obtained through multiple-choice questions.

---

**TABLE 4-7. Goals Statement from a Student Paper Interviewing the Mother of the Child-Patient**

P: Mother's verbalized goals include
1. He will be able to pick up food with a fork or spoon and be able to eat independently.
2. He will be able to drink from a cup independently and not play with the cup or turn it over.
*3. The patient's twin will become involved in the last 5 minutes of the therapy sessions at _____ Hospital to the degree that the twin won't mimic the patient in order to obtain attention.

Verbalization of goals was at the open-ended level of participation.

*Primary goal.

---

**TABLE 4-8. Student-Written SOAP Note Based on Work with an Aphasic Patient**

**S:** Patient has expressive aphasia but was able to indicate 3 concerns in response to an open-ended question by pointing to the area troubling him.

Patient indicated that he had trouble with his right arm, with his right leg, and with his hearing. Indicated that his greatest concern was his right leg, but when checking out, patient indicated he wanted to work on his hearing problem first.

**O:**

**A:**

**P:** Patient goals were elicited through multiple-choice questions. Most important goal specified on level of concurrence.
1. to understand what people say better
*2. be able to understand what people are saying when they talk fast to the degree that he can follow directions
3. be able to let people know to slow down when talking

*Most important goal.

question as to what else he would like to do. He spoke on his own; he said, "I want to go home."

**Therapist:** What do you need to do in order to go home?
**Patient:** Get up.
**Therapist:** Anything else?
**Patient:** Walk.
**Therapist:** Ok, let me help you get up. (The patient assisted me in getting him to a sitting position on the edge of the bed. He sat there for about a minute with his feet close to the floor.)
**Therapist:** Are you ready to walk?
**Patient:** (Nods yes.)
**Therapist:** How far would you like to walk this time? (When he did not respond for several seconds, I said) Let me offer you some suggestions: Would you like to walk 2 feet, 5 feet, or 10 feet?
**Patient:** Five feet.
**Therapist:** OK, let's try to walk the 5 feet. (Patient walks in a shuffling fashion, one foot after the other, for a total of 5 steps toward the other bed in his room.)
**Therapist:** That was well done. You walked 5 feet as you wanted. Are you ready to walk any further?
**Patient:** No. (I helped him back to his bed and helped him lie down.)
**Therapist:** You accomplished the 5 feet you set out to walk. What helped you to do that?
**Patient:** (Points to me and starts to cry but stops himself.)
**Therapist:** Is there anyone else or anything else that helped you walk? Let me give you some suggestions. It was you telling me what you wanted, it was you moving your feet, it was you saying how far you wanted to walk. Any of those things that you did that helped?
**Patient:** Me telling you what I wanted.
**Therapist:** It helped when you told me what you wanted. Tomorrow when I come to work with you again, I'd like you to tell me what you want to do and I'll try to do it with you.

Flexibility is also needed with patients with special problems in communication. Tables 4–7 and 4–8 are examples of how the format can be used successfully with children and with aphasic patients. Because of communication problems, the patient in Table 4–8 was unable to answer open-ended questions regarding concerns. The student therefore started with multiple choice, and the patient was able to shake his head yes or no to the ideas offered.

# Section
# *two*

The knowledge and skills needed to involve patients in a meaningful way in their own therapeutic program planning has been presented in the first four chapters. Emphasis has been on an interpersonal process and an attitudinal mind set that are applicable to a wide variety of patients, rather than on knowledge and skills related to diagnostic categories or treatment modalities. Both are essential for professional problem solving. We have detailed our model of a treatment plan, consisting of *goals*, *means*, and *time line*. We have recommended questions and the sequencing of questions that will enable the reader to lead the patient through the process. We have recommended that, ultimately, the patient should be taught to lead himself or herself through the process and thus become a more independent, self-reliant problem solver relative to his or her own problems. We have encouraged the process personally before teaching it to others, to model roles in the process and to understand it experientially as well as intellectually.

This second section deals with the generalization of the techniques described within Section One. Rather than how therapists can apply techniques to themselves in learning how to master this approach to planning, Chapter 5 describes how therapists can use this planning technique throughout their professional development. One may also begin to understand the use of the planning questions with patient groups, as well as with individual patients. As in relation to one's work with individual patients, it is important to recognize the opportunity to learn to master such techniques by experiencing it oneself as a member of a group. A classroom can serve to provide such an experience. Chapter 6 thus describes 2 different models for conducting such group-based training. The academic course illustrates application throughout an undergraduate program in several phases, geared to the rest of the student's professional development and thus integrated into the entire curriculum. The in-service model is more time limited, with focus on immediate

**63**

clinical application in a relatively efficient manner. This last chapter thus describes the details of the means of achieving the goals and objectives set out originally in Chapter 1.

# 5

# *Further*
# *Applications*

Thus far, there has been a focus on the relationship between the individual patient/client and a therapist and in learning how to use this approach with patients by first using it in this course for oneself. Answering the planning questions through the steps of exploration, selection, and specification can also be used in other situations. This section will illustrate the application of these questions and steps to different educational settings in the professional life of the therapist. This chapter also aims to introduce the reader to application of the patient-participation-in-planning model in a group setting. Addressing these same questions and going through the process of answering them in a group setting require some modification of the procedures used up to now.

## PROFESSIONAL GROWTH AND DEVELOPMENT

Beginning with formal professional education, therapists are thrust into a lifelong educational process. Stimuli for this continuing education are both external and internal. External stimuli include licensure requirements, agency policies, collegial exchanges, and challenging patient cases. Internal stimuli arise from a recognition of a gap in one's knowledge; that more information on a topic is needed to feel competent.

To learn efficiently, it is helpful to utilize a structured process. The planning method described in this book provides such a structure. One can choose to use form PPS–1W (W for *weighting*), a modification of PPS–1, to explore concerns relative to the topic of interest and to select a major concern. A

**65**

shared weighting procedure is used for the selection step in respect to concerns. This shared weighting procedure has been described in Chapter 2. One can then explore goals and specify a goal. The PPS–1W form illustrated in Table 5–1, adds a section for *value* of concerns, which is determined by the shared weighting process.

The following are examples of the process being used to establish learning goals. In the first situation, senior occupational therapy students were each asked to submit to the instructor three topic choices for a term paper. The instructor then reviewed the topics, approved one, and returned the selected topic to each student. However, many of the students had difficulty selecting three choices to submit. Table 5–2 demonstrates the use of the planning process to arrive at a topic by one student. Note that she arrived at a major concern of not knowing enough about diagnoses through the shared weighting process; this concern had a value of 4 for her. As a part of her specific goal, she felt that her referral in her paper to data from between 5 and 10 articles on the topic of psychosocial aspects of spinal cord injury would be a measure of having met her goal. In other cases, one might consider using 5–10 articles to be a means by which she might meet a goal of understanding psychosocial aspects.

In a second example, a postprofessional graduate student used the procedure as she neared the completion of her degree. The process enabled the student to identify a goal relative to future clinical work. The results are presented in Table 5–3. For two of her concerns statements, she elected to make multiple comments for the purpose of clarification. For example, she clarified in concern statement 1.B that she had a specific problem with the differential diagnosis of wrist and pain disorders. Use of these multiple comments as part of exploration may be very helpful to a user of the process. Also, note that the student expressed 4 goals rather than 3. Three steps of exploration are considered a reasonable minimum; more items are permissible if the person chooses.

In a third situation, a postprofessional graduate student had completed the first phase of a teaching practicum and was preparing for the second phase. To help the student prepare for the next phase, PPS–1W was used. Table 5–4 summarizes the results. Following the completion of the second and final phase, PPS–3 was used. The PPS–3 results are illustrated in Table 5–5.

You the reader can use the planning process for your own continuing self-education. Perhaps you have to research a difficult patient case. Or perhaps you have to organize and present a department in-service program. Use the blank PPS–1W (Table 5–1) form provided to begin to address whatever educational concerns you have just as you have done throughout this book.

---

**TABLE 5-1.  PPS-1W**

---

NAME _____                    DATE _____

1. **What are your concerns?**
   A.
   B.
   C.

2. **What are your major concerns?**
*Values*
   A.
   B.
   C.

3. **What do you want to see happen? What would make you feel that you are making progress? What are your goals? Choose one.**
   A.
   B.
   C.

4. **What is your specific goal?**

   | A | B | C | D | **What?** |
   | A | B | C | D | **Conditions?** |
   | A | B | C | D | **Degree?** |

   A = open-ended question: FREE CHOICE
   B = suggestions (3 options): MULTIPLE CHOICE
   C = recommendation (1 option): FORCED CHOICE
   D = prescription (tell what to do): NO CHOICE

---

**TABLE 5-2. PPS-1W: Selection of Paper Topic**

1. **What are your concerns?**
   A. Patient transfers
   B. Not knowing diagnoses well enough to intervene with patients
   C. Evaluations-time lapse since learning evaluations such as joint range of motion and muscle testing

2. **What are your major concerns?**
   *Values*

   | | | | | |
   |---|---|---|---|---|
   | (2) | 1 | | 1 | A. Patient transfers |
   | (4) | | 2 | 2 | B. Not knowing diagnoses well enough to intervene with patients |
   | (3) | 2 | 1 | | C. Evaluations-time lapse since learning evaluations such as joint range of motion and muscle testing |

3. **What do you want to see happen? What would make you feel that you are making progress? What are your goals? Choose one.**
   A. With CVA patients, knowing where to start, what to do first, what kind of activities to use
   *B. With SCI patients, knowing where to start
   C. With head injury patients, knowing where to start

4. **What is your specific goal?**

   **What?**      I want to be able to discuss psychosocial aspects of spinal cord injury and its implications for occupational therapy,
   **Conditions?**      in a paper,
   **Degree?**      discussing 5-10 articles.

**Time line:** November 11, paper due date

---

# GROUP APPLICATIONS

Therapists are frequently required to lead groups, whether they are patient therapy groups, professional planning groups, or educational groups. The purpose of this section is to introduce how the basic ideas for patient participation in planning can be used to run a group. Since group methods and dynamics are not an emphasis of this book, we are not addressing them in detail. Following a general discussion of the application of the planning process to groups, an example of its use in running a patient group is presented.

## GROUP PROCEDURES

The procedures in leading a group are essentially the same as those used with the patient in the clinical setting. In answering each of the questions, it

---

**TABLE 5-3. PPS-1W: Graduate Student Interview**

1. **What are your concerns?**
   A. Schedule of 2 patients per hour with instantaneous decisions needed; need to be able to make quick judgments
   B. Differential diagnosis; especially with pain and wrist disorders
   C. Don't trust my sensory mapping with the Semmes-Weinstein

2. **What are your major concerns?**
   *Values*

   | | | | | |
   |---|---|---|---|---|
   | (5) | 3 | 2 | A. | Schedule of 2 patients per hour with instantaneous decisions needed; need to be able to make quick judgments |
   | (3) | | 2 | 1 | B. Differential diagnosis; especially with pain and wrist disorders |
   | (1) | 0 | 1 | C. | Don't trust my sensory mapping with the Semmes-Weinstein |

3. **What do you want to see happen? What would make you feel that you are making progress? What are your goals? Choose one.**
   *A. Less second guessing about treatment after the patient has left
   B. Less anxiety prior to patient visits
   C. Less need to consult books before making a decision
   D. Send the patient out knowing that I've done my best

4. **What is your specific goal?**

   **What?**  I want to utilize all appropriate therapeutic principles (e.g., splinting) to their optimal levels

   **Conditions?**  with persons with new hand injuries at the time of their first clinic visit

   **Degree?**  75% of the time.

**Time line:** If working 20 hours/week, by February 1

---

is necessary to perform the steps of exploration, selection, and specification but now in a group setting. The exploration step follows the model of "brainstorming," in which judgment is deferred. Such deferral of judgment during exploration serves to encourage as much input as possible from the group members. The number of ideas listed by the group should be in the range of more than 2 per person. In a group of 10–12 persons, one would aim for exploration to encompass in the range of 30 statements.

It is possible for participants even in a group as large as 35 or more to be allowed to speak for themselves. Participants are asked to volunteer their concerns, and efforts are made to encourage as many as possible to participate. As the ideas are placed on the chalkboard or easel paper, there is no judgment. Neither positive nor negative statements are made about the quality of the ideas. The exploration step requires that all the concerns be ex-

---

**TABLE 5-4.  PPS-1W: Preparing for Teaching Practicum**

1. **What are your concerns?**
   A.  Frustration over students not understanding what is being said in lecture
   B.  My lecture delivery may not be interesting—too flat?
   C.  I'd like to balance my presentation with handouts and other varied learning experiences.

2. **What are your major concerns?**
   *Values*

   | | | | | |
   |---|---|---|---|---|
   | (4) | 2 | | 2 | A.  Frustration over students not understanding what is being said in lecture |
   | (2) | | 1 | 1 | B.  My lecture delivery may not be interesting—too flat? |
   | (3) | 1 | | 2 | C.  I'd like to balance my presentation with handouts and other varied learning experiences |

3. **What do you want to see happen? What would make you feel that you are making progress? What are your goals? Choose one.**
   A.  Students will be able to do the lab exercise correctly without asking questions.
   *B. I will see that the students are doing the lab exercises correctly.
   C.  Students will independently ask questions while indicating that they have integrated information.

4. **What is your specific goal?**
   **What?**           I would like to present the basic technique of proprioceptive neuromuscular facilitation
   **Conditions?**     in 2-hour lecture/labs October 18 and 20
   **Degree?**         so that students complete all exercises according to the guidelines established in the syllabus.

---

pressed before they are responded to or before further selection or specification. The deferral of judgment and the acceptance of the level of specificity of the ideas as initially stated encourages group members to speak out. After many have spoken, each participant who has not spoken freely can be asked his or her concerns. The participant may also choose to select from those ideas already listed by others (multiple choice). It is important that persons be encouraged to state their own version of the ideas they have selected. It has been our experience that each person's ideas differ somewhat in detail.

A preassignment that requires group members to address the exploration of concerns or any of the other questions may be used when working with large groups or where there are other time constraints. Thus, participants

**TABLE 5-5. PPS-3: Teaching Practicum**

1. **What results have you achieved?**
   A. Didn't complete in 2 hours as planned but did present all I wanted to
   B. More comfortable with using slides and overhead projector
   *C. Students followed the guidelines in the syllabus completing the lab exercises correctly about proprioceptive neuromuscular facilitation in lecture/lab on October 18 and 20

2. **What worked?**
   A. Newness motivated them
   B. I reminded them to refer to the syllabus guidelines
   C. Used more slides

3. **What are your concerns?**
   *Values*

| | | | | |
|---|---|---|---|---|
| (4) | 2 | | 2 | A. Balance amount of information and time frame |
| (3) | | 2 | 1 | B. My lecture pace was too fast |
| (2) | 1 | 1 | | C. Lack of immediate student feedback |

4. **Goals**
   * A. Provide same content without extending beyond 2-hour limit
   B. Sense that information is presented in an integrated fashion
   C. Students performing more independently in lab

5. **What is plan?**
   **Goal:** Present same content on neuromuscular facilitation in next session within 2-hour time limit
   **Means:** Using 25–30 colored slides during presentation to graduate students depicting diagonals of motion, combined movements of upper and lower extremities, and basic procedures

   **Time line:** By the end of spring semester

may individually perform the appropriate steps in the process and then share their answers in the group setting.

The selection step in a group can also be handled so as to take advantage of the group format. One may form subgroups which could be asked to "cluster" the ideas already listed. One may ask each small group to list 3-5 categories that would encompass all the ideas listed in the exploration step. This clustering procedure permits the retention of the original variety of ideas but in a more manageable way. One can thus establish a group consensus by finding similarities in the clusters developed by each of the small groups.

Another format for selection from a large list generated during the exploration step is to have individual group members select three important concerns from those generated by the entire group. These selected concerns can then be used by the participants to have weights or values applied. The following is an example of a group member's selection of concerns from the list generated by the group. She then applied paired weighting with 3 points to be split between the items in each pair to determine her major concern. (The figures in parentheses refer to the weights).

(3)  Not able to spend time on goal setting when first beginning therapy
(4)  Setting appropriate time lines for the goals
(2)  Writing goals that can be reimbursed by insurers

Each group member then converted his or her selection of the highest priority concern into a goal statement. The single highest priority goal from each was amalgamated into a list by the leader, thus identifying the goals of the entire group. Such a list was generated by a group of occupational therapy graduate students (with the figures in parentheses referring to the number of times each goal was stated):

---

**TABLE 5–6. Inservice, Session 1**

*Exploration* of group concerns of involving patients in program planning
1. Cognitive status, concerns pre vs post injury
2. How much can they be involved; abstraction; short-term and long-term carry-over after discharge
3. Follow-through after discharge
4. Depression and denial interferes with motivation to accomplish goals
5. If patient denies, will he plan treatment
6. If patient included, therapist not doing job
7. Patient fear of interacting with professionals
8. Overachievers may set unrealistic goals
9. Newly disabled—long time to realize what goals are possible
10. For old disabled—long time to realize what goals are possible
11. Professionals would have to change attitude toward patient
12. What if patient's goal doesn't correspond with M.D.'s goal?
13. With children, goal setting and communication with family is a problem
14. Difficult setting goals with changing status—deteriorating or improving
15. Overburdening parents with therapy responsibility
16. Involving those in goal setting who want to be left alone
17. Time elements and relationship—takes time to achieve, especially in acute care
18. Find out the reason they're unmotivated (e.g., pain, failure)
19. Is it realistic that patient and therapist do all goal setting without M.D.
20. Financial obligations keep patients from setting goals and attending therapy

---

**TABLE 5-7. Clustering of Data from Exploration of Concerns in Table 5-6**

---

*Realistic goals:* Overachievers set unrealistic goals; newly disabled may not realize what is possible; old disabled may require long time to realize what goals are possible; if patient denies, will he plan treatment?

*Cognitively impaired:* Cognitive status, concerns pre vs post injury; how much can they be involved, abstraction, short-term and long-term carry-over after discharge?

*Motivation:* Follow through after discharge; depression and denial interfere with motivation to accomplish goals; find out the reason they're unmotivated (e.g., pain, failure); involving those in goal setting who want to be left alone

*Patient, Family, and Professional Relationships:* If patient included, therapist not doing job; patient fear of interacting with professionals; professionals would have to change attitude toward patient; what if patient's goal doesn't correspond with M.D.'s goal; with children, goal setting and communication with family is a problem; overburdening parents with therapy responsibility; time elements and relationship—takes time to achieve, especially in acute care; is it realistic that patient and therapist do all goal setting without M.D.?

---

(8)  Establish priorities for goals
(6)  Set appropriate time lines for review, such as immediately, 3 months, and so forth
(4)  Write patient goals that meet the individual's needs; respect patient's cultures and beliefs
(3)  Patient will participate in goals that are set primarily by the therapist as well as in those arising primarily from the patient
(3)  Goals will be reimbursable by third-party payment

Still another alternative is for the group leader to perform selection for the group by clustering the concerns. Common themes among the concerns are identified, and specific comments that support each major category are grouped along with the theme of the category. Tables 5–6 and 5–7 describe both the exploration and the selection via clusters for material generated during the first session in an in-service program for both physical and occupational therapists. These clusters then served as a basis for generating goals for this course.

Form PPS–1G (*G* for *group*), a modified version of PPS–1, has been developed to use with groups. It helps one organize a group's concerns, the major concerns via clustering, and general goals. Table 5–8 is a blank PPS–1G provided for the use of the reader.

---

**TABLE 5–8. PPS–1G**

1. What are the group's concerns (identify average of 2–3 for each participant)?
   A.
   B.
   C.
   •
   •
   Z.

2. What are the group's major concerns? Identify 3–4 major themes from the list of group concerns and list relevant concerns after each theme (clustering). Have group select by either ranking or by weighting.

   Value A. Theme _____ :
       B. Theme _____ :
       C. Theme _____ :
       D. Theme _____ :

3. What does the group want to see happen? What would indicate to the group that it's making progress with the top ranked or weighted cluster? Explore and list.
   A.
   B.
   •
   •
   Z.

---

The specification step can also be done on a group basis by involving the other members of the group in providing suggestions (multiple choice) for the particular person who is being asked to specify a statement. The group leader could also serve as a source of ideas, but it is preferable for the fellow group members to serve as a resource. The leader or the group members must model the process to be followed by asking permission before moving from free choice to multiple choice and so forth. As the group becomes more familiar with the steps and the use of the various questions, the leader can encourage the group members to assume the role of questioners during the sessions.

## Application to a Patient Group

One of the major concerns in the management of persons with spinal cord injury is the need for hospitalization for relatively long periods for the treatment of skin breakdown. In dealing with this problem, a "skin care support group" was designed in the model of patient participation in planning. This illustrates the application of the principles of maximal patient participation in answering several of the planning questions in a group, with emphasis on the exploration phase. Since the topic addressed was that of prevention of skin breakdown, the problem was defined as *"What are some causes for skin breakdown?"* The question was posed on the easel board by the staff group leader. Exploration was performed by the group answering the question freely on their own. The staff did not offer ideas unless there were none forthcoming. It was rarely necessary to offer any ideas because each of the persons had problems with skin breakdown and could deal with his or her own experiences as to what might cause such problems. The staff leader was responsible for encouraging input from all members of the group, and no judgment was made as to whether ideas were "good" or "bad." Each idea was recognized by having it placed on the easel board, thus giving evidence of its having been heard. It was thus also possible for the person stating the idea to be certain that it was being heard properly. During the exploration phase, at least 15–20 statements would surface in a group of 6–8 patients.

Once the exploration phase ended, the selection step was carried out by the group to identify the 3 most important causes or problems. A voting procedure was used wherein each of the members identified what he or she thought was the most important cause. The causes getting the most votes were then used for the next phase. For each of the problems so identified, the question *"What would work to deal with this problem?"* was posed on the easel board. During this exploration phase 3 solutions were again elicited in answer to each of the problems.

It was considered important that the persons with problems begin to think of possible solutions. The threefold exploration of possible solutions was a method to develop a sense of possibility of alternatives. For example, one of the causes for skin breakdown was "sitting too long." The solutions generated were such as "remembering to shift weight," "lifting up," "paying attention to a burning feeling." If fewer than 3 possible solutions arose freely from the group, the professional serving as facilitator would offer several choices from ideas mentioned by other patients in the past. However, the ideas were not listed on the easel board unless spoken by one of the members of the group.

At the end of each of these 45-minute sessions, the group members were then asked to evaluate the activity just completed. The questions "*What happened in the group? What results occurred?*" were posed. After having elicited possible outcomes, the question "*What did we do that helped to bring about those results?*" was asked. Out of this evaluation came ideas as to how to improve and expand the sessions. An example of the answers as to outcome were such statements as "I learned something new that I could use." Among the ideas listed in answer to what worked, the members of the group made such statements as "getting help from others," "hearing what other people know."

The effects of these sessions were evaluated in terms of reduced incidence of skin breakdown in these persons and by several other parameters relevant to the management of persons with spinal cord injury. The issue for emphasis is that the ideas were not in themselves new. What was new was the opportunity for the persons with the problem to be the ones speaking about it. Not only could they speak about their problems but they also could take part in their solutions and have a role in evaluating what was being done in the sessions.

Still other sessions in this same format dealt with other aspects that would lead to reduction in the severity and frequency of pressure sores. A second session dealt with early identification of skin breakdown if it did occur. The question as to concerns was phrased "How would you know you have a pressure sore?" The group members specified their answers to that question in terms of not only *what* was looked for but also *where* and *when*. For example, the several answers to *what* was looked for included "redness," "softening of skin," "hard spot," and "drying." Following this, the next question dealt with what could be done once one identified a problem. One is thus dealing with the question "*What works?*"

As a result of this program, significant changes occurred in the frequency and severity of skin ulcers in this group of patients, who had been hospitalized for quite long periods in the past. In reviewing with those patients some months later the methods that may have contributed to these changes, many of their comments related to the content of the sessions and the ideas that they heard about that worked. Several patients also specified the ways that the sessions had been conducted as useful. For example, one aspect mentioned was the fact that they were asked to look at different answers to the question and not just one. One man described it as follows: "We had a chance to get different perspectives. There was no right or wrong answer but we had a chance to think about things." He went on to say that he used this approach in relation to many other problems he had in dealing with his life since he had learned about it in the skin care group.

# 6

# *Educational Programs*

To learn the planning process in a group setting such as a classroom provides an opportunity once again for the student/therapist to experience in a personal way the same procedures eventually used with patients. The ultimate aim is to integrate the procedures illustrated in this book into the future professional life of the therapist/ student. This chapter describes in detail a formal academic course and an in-service training course.

## ACADEMIC COURSE

This course dealt with the entire set of questions for undergraduate students over the length of their educational program throughout their first full year in professional school. Some assignments connected with the course were integrated into the schedule of the various types of field assignments.

Patient participation in planning was the first unit of a course entitled "Clinical Problem Solving and Communications." This course took place during the first semester for entering undergraduate physical therapy students and was generally concerned with the following goals: to provide models for clinical problem solving, interpersonal communications, and ethical decision making; and to discuss psychosocial issues that influence those three models. The participatory planning process is perceived to be related to all 3 functions.

The goals of this initial participatory planning component are to lead each student to experience the specification of concerns and goals for self, with peers, and with a patient. The unit begins with several lectures and laboratories on the 2 basic questions outlined in Chapter 2. It ends with the students carrying out an interview with one patient, eliciting specific goals in an area relevant to concerns, with maximal patient participation. This is critiqued by faculty and peers using a standard evaluation form (Table 6–1). We have made several videotapes of patients being interviewed so that the students can have an example to critique using a standard scoring form (Table 6–2). The students are introduced to the third planning question in dealing with evaluation of outcomes immediately after the completion of this first patient interview, and they set new goals for themselves. This patient interview is their first experience in clinical interaction within the entire curriculum. The class then proceeds to other topics.

We return to participatory patient planning 3 further times with assignments for fall and spring part-time clinical work and prior to their full-time summer clinical affiliation between their first and second curricular years. The goals for these later assignments are as follows. For the fall clinical rotation, the students apply the experience doing the supervised interview to 2 additional patients, on their own. They deal with the questions of concerns and goals in the clinical setting. The spring rotation provides an opportunity to see a patient more than once, so the students are asked to interview the same patient more than once and to ask the question about outcomes and reevaluation of concerns and goals in the light of those outcomes. Further, they integrate the results of these interviews into the clinical record (SOAP notes or narrative). This material is incorporated in Chapter 4. The summer affiliation provides an opportunity to follow at least 1 patient over several weeks. The assignment from this course is for the first time to document all 5 questions in the format of the medical record. A detailed curricular plan for this entire program follows.

## OUTLINE OF AN UNDERGRADUATE COURSE FOR PHYSICAL THERAPY STUDENTS IN PATIENT PARTICIPATION IN PLANNING

The first part of this course can be done in approximately 6 weeks, with one lecture and one laboratory each week, as indicated below.

I. Session 1: 50 minutes (large group)
   A. Preclass activities
      1. Prepare syllabus for the course (schedule, topical outline, reading assignments, reprints, and so forth).
   B. Classroom activities
      1. Outline the entire course on clinical problem solving and communications.

**TABLE 6–1. Interview Evaluation Form: Patient Participation in Planning for Therapy**

| | Not Attempted | Attempted | | Comments |
|---|---|---|---|---|
| | | Incomplete | Complete | |
| 1. Did interviewer<br> A. introduce patient to overall procedures?<br> B. introduce exploration of concerns?<br> C. elicit at least 3 concerns?<br> D. ask for selection of priorities (either shared weights or priority)?<br> E. confirm major concern(s)?<br> F. introduce exploration of goals?<br> G. introduce cooperative role in identifying goals?<br> H. elicit 3 goals?<br> I. ask for selection of one goal to pursue?<br> J. specify goal: what?<br> K. setting?<br> L. degree?<br>2. Did interview start with open-ended question?<br>3. Did interviewer ask patient's consent before moving to multiple choice, forced choice, or prescription?<br>4. Did student move down steps in correct order?<br>5. Did student return to open-ended questions at an appropriate time? | | | | |

**TABLE 6–2. Scoring Form for Analysis of Videotapes**

| The Therapist | 1 | 2 | 3 | 4 | 5 | 6 | 7 | 8 | 9 | 10 | 11 | 12 | 13 | 14 | 15 |
|---|---|---|---|---|---|---|---|---|---|---|---|---|---|---|---|
| A. Asks open-ended questions without suggesting answers | | | | | | | | | | | | | | | |
| B. Suggests 3 options/answers | | | | | | | | | | | | | | | |
| C. Recommends 1 option/answer | | | | | | | | | | | | | | | |
| D. Tells what to do | | | | | | | | | | | | | | | |
| E. Reflection and Other | | | | | | | | | | | | | | | |

| | 16 | 17 | 18 | 19 | 20 | 21 | 22 | 23 | 24 | 25 | 26 | 27 | 28 | 29 | 30 |
|---|---|---|---|---|---|---|---|---|---|---|---|---|---|---|---|
| A. Asks open-ended questions without suggesting answers | | | | | | | | | | | | | | | |
| B. Suggests 3 options/answers | | | | | | | | | | | | | | | |
| C. Recommends 1 option/answer | | | | | | | | | | | | | | | |
| D. Tells what to do | | | | | | | | | | | | | | | |
| E. Reflection and Other | | | | | | | | | | | | | | | |

      2. Make an assignment to read the Introduction and Chapter 1 in this book.

  C. Instructional aids

      1. Textbook

      2. Course syllabus

      3. Chalkboard

II. Session 2: 50 minutes (large group)

  A. Preclass activities

      1. Prepare extra copies of PPS–1.

  B. Classroom activities

      1. Review and expand on instructor's concerns that led to the development of this course and the instructor's goals for the course.

      2. Ask, "What are your concerns?" Lecture, stimulate discussion of the content of assigned text. Illustrate use of the exercise at the end of Chapter 1.

      3. Ask as many students as time allows to state their concerns about mastering the knowledge and skills taught in this segment of this course. Write their concerns on the board.

      4. Hand out additional copies of PPS–1 and ask the students to complete it relative to *their own* concerns in this course, to be completed before their first laboratory. Assign Chapter 2 in the text.

  C. Instructional aids

      1. Handouts (PPS–1)

      2. Chalkboard

III. Session 3: 2 hours, in groups of 10 students or less

  A. Laboratory exercise

      1. Each student states his or her chief concern from the PPS–1 forms. These concerns are written on the board, and one student acts as secretary to record on paper what is written on the board. The instructor saves this paper for use in the next laboratory.

      2. Each student then specifies (what, where or when, and degree) his or her own concern.

      3. As opportunity or need arises, instruction and examples are provided by the instructor on any course-relevant points raised by the exercise.

      4. Hand out additional copies of PPS–1 and ask the students to complete it in its entirety in terms of concerns, goals, and specificity of goals to be completed before next large group session.

  B. Instructional aids

      1. Chalkboard

      2. Paper and pencil

IV. Session 4: 50 minutes (large group)

A. Preclass activities
  1. Prepare handout of PPS-1.
B. Classroom activities
  1. Opportunity for students to state their concerns on previous learning activities is provided.
  2. Lecture, discuss, and illustrate content relative to goals.
  3. As time permits, write a few student-generated goals on the board from the student's homework assignments, emphasizing specificity of goals.
  4. Discuss and illustrate differences between goals and means.
  5. Hand out a copy of PPS-1 and assign student to interview someone (e.g., relative, friend) other than a classmate using this form and to complete the concerns and goals portion of the form; due in 1 week.
C. Instructional aids
  1. PPS-1
  2. Chalkboard
V. Session 5: 2 hours, in groups of 10 students or less
  A. Prelaboratory activities
    1. Arrange for video equipment to be in the laboratory.
    2. Evaluate PPS-1 homework assignments and return.
  B. Laboratory exercise
    1. Each student reads his or her chief concern from the record made in the first laboratory exercise. The student then states a goal for that concern, and the goal is written on the board. The student specifies his or her goal. Students are encouraged to ask for assistance from other class members, if necessary. Class members can also ask for permission to offer suggestions.
    2. A videotape of a patient interview done by one of the instructors is shown. The tape should be stopped frequently by the instructor to illustrate and discuss what is happening in the taped interview, emphasizing the levels of participation and the fact that the interviewer informed the patient of what was to happen and asked permission to move down the scale of levels of participation used in Table 2-1.
    3. As opportunity or need arises, instruction and examples should be provided by the instructor on any course-relevant points raised by the exercise.
  C. Instructional aids
    1. Chalkboard
    2. Videotaped interview
    3. Videotape player and screen
VI. Session 6: 50 minutes (large group)
  A. Preclass activities
    1. Prepare at least 4 copies for each student of handouts of a scor-

ing sheet based on Table 2–1.
2. Read and comment on PPS–1 forms from peer interviews; return through student mailboxes.
3. Prepare a schedule for clinical interviews.
B. Classroom activities
1. Opportunity to express concerns on previous learning activities is provided. What outcomes were achieved? What problems remain?
2. Lecture, discuss, and illustrate content relative to scoring interviews for levels of patient participation.
3. Discuss the videotape quiz scheduled for next week. Hand out and discuss the scoring form.
4. Hand out and discuss schedule of clinical interviews.
C. Instructional aids
1. Handouts or videotape scoring form and interview schedule.
VII. Session 7: 2 hours, with groups of 10 students or less
A. Prelaboratory activities
1. Arrange for videotape equipment to be in the laboratory.
2. Arrange to place videotapes in media library for student use.
B. Laboratory exercise
1. A videotape of an interview done by an instructor is viewed with frequent interruptions to discuss level of patient participation illustrated in the interview. Students score.
2. Students view a second taped interview and score without interruption. Students then compare their scoring efforts, and the laboratory project is discussed.
3. Students are offered the opportunity to study videotapes of interviews in the media library of the university.
C. Instructional aids
1. Scoring forms for video interviews (Table 6–2)
2. Videotapes of two interviews
3. Video equipment
VIII. Session 8: 30 minutes (large group), videotape quiz.
A. Preclass activities
1. Have available a videotaped interview that the students have not seen.
2. Prepare handouts of patient participation scoring forms.
3. Arrange for videotape viewing equipment to be in the classroom.
B. Classroom activities
1. Hand out patient participation scoring forms.
2. Show videotaped interview for students to score.
C. Instructional aids
1. Videotaped interview
2. Videotape-viewing equipment

   3. Scoring forms
   D. Postquiz activity
   1. Grade quiz and report scores to students in some appropriate way.
IX. Session 9: 45 minutes for *each* student, in groups of 3 or 4 students per instructor
   A. Preclinical activity
   1. Prepare sufficient copies of form PPS–1.
   2. Prepare sufficient copies of form found in Table 6–1.
   3. Schedule patients and students.
   B. Clinical activities
   1. Each student interviews a patient, working from PPS–1 to obtain all information required by that form.
   2. Other students and instructor fill out form from Table 6–1.
   3. Interviewing student critiques himself or herself and discusses his or her interview.
   4. Each observing student provides feedback to the interviewing student concerning his or her performance during the interview.
   5. The instructor provides feedback to the interviewing student and makes such other instructional points as may have been illustrated during the interview. The interviews are not graded, because our experience indicates that grading creates such anxiety that little learning occurs.

   The 9 sessions outlined above constitute a unit within the year-long course on clinical problem solving and communications. It occupies about 6 weeks. Other units are taken up in sequence after Session 9. The following sessions are interspersed at appropriate times during the year.

X. Session 10: fall part-time clinical experience
   A. Assignment: 15 minutes (large group)
   1. Students are given form PPS–2 and asked to fill it out and hand it in to the instructor before beginning the fall clinical rotation of a half a day per week for 2 weeks. It is to be completed in regard to *their own* accomplishments, remaining concerns and goals in completing their own learning or knowledge, and skills relative to the content of this book.
   B. Preclinical activities
   1. Critique student forms PPS–2 in terms of threefold exploration and specification of selected outcomes, concerns, and goals. Return to students prior to their clinical rotation.
   2. Hand out form PPS–1 and assign students to complete the form with at least 1 patient during their fall clinical rotation and turn it in to the instructor.

    C. Postclinical activities

       1. Critique student forms PPS–1 done during the clinical rotation with particular emphasis on relevance of goals to selected main concern, adequate exploration of goals, specification of selected goal, and level of participation. Return them to students.

XI. Session 11: spring part-time clinical experience

    A. Assignment: 15 minutes (large group)

       1. Students are given form PPS–3 and asked to fill it out and hand it in to the instructor before beginning the spring clinical rotation of 1 full day per week for 2 weeks. It is to be completed in regard to *their own* concerns in completing their learning or knowledge and skills relative to the content of this book.

       2. Read Chapter 3 in textbook.

    B. Preclinical activities

       1. Critique student forms PPS–3 and return to students prior to their clinical rotation.

       2. Hand out forms PPS–1 and PPS–2 and assign students to complete both the initial and follow-up forms with a patient during their spring clinical rotation and to turn it in to the instructor. Hand in copies of their clinical SOAP notes containing material relevant to this course.

       3. Discuss in class the content of Chapter 3, emphasizing the question of outcomes. (15 minutes [large group])

    C. Postclinical activities

       1. Critique student forms and SOAP notes written during the clinical rotation with same emphasis as in the fall clinical rotation and return them to students.

XII. Session 12: summer full-time clinical affiliation

    A. Assignment: 15 minutes (large group)

       1. Students are given form PPS–3 and asked to fill it out and hand it in to the instructor before beginning the summer clinical rotation. It is to be completed in regard to *their own* concerns in completing their learning or knowledge and skills relative to the content of this book.

       2. Read Chapter 4 in textbook.

    B. Preclinical activities

       1. Critique student forms PPS–3, which should be complete in every respect, and return to students prior to their clinical rotation.

       2. Discuss in class the content of Chapter 4, emphasizing the question of what worked. (30 minutes [large group])

       3. Assign the students to hand in at the end of the summer one SOAP note (or whatever format is used in the clinic where they work). This copy of the clinical record is to demonstrate the answering of all 5 questions posed in the Introduction to this

text. It must, therefore, represent at least 3 evaluative sessions with the patient.
C. Postclinical activities
   1. Critique student SOAP notes or other documentation done during the clinical rotation and return to students.

# IN-SERVICE TRAINING

A short-term course for physical and occupational therapists in a large medical center used the planning process as a basis for its organization as well as for its content. The staff supervisors felt that there was a need for the staff to meet the requirements of accreditation agencies to incorporate patients into the planning process to a greater degree. Still other issues dealt with staff burnout and the need to develop new formats for working with the large variety of patients, particularly those with cognitive impairments. The concerns of the therapists themselves have been illustrated earlier in Table 5–6. They formed the basis for the design of the course to be described.

The course lasted 7 hours and was implemented in conjunction with the daily duties of the therapists and was applied in their own work. Once the therapists had experienced the first 2 questions as to concerns and goals and the awareness of the levels of participation, they put these several questions to work with patients.

By the end of the course, the classroom sessions had dealt with the entire set of questions. Once the therapists had experienced the use of the questions in the classroom, they then applied them to their work with patients. Emphasis was primarily on the steps of exploration, selection, and specification and levels of participation as exemplified in any one or several of the questions. The specific goals of each of the sessions, the procedures followed, and the evaluation of results are described in detail as follows.

## IN-SERVICE COURSE: PATIENT PARTICIPATION IN PROGRAM PLANNING—OCCUPATIONAL AND PHYSICAL THERAPY DEPARTMENTS

### Instructor's Course Goal (Outcome)

**What:** participants will be able to generate outcome statements, solution statements, need statements, and goal statements
**When/where:** during the course of ongoing therapeutic relationship daily or as needed

**Degree:** meeting the criteria of specificity, relevance, and fit as appropriate for the content of the statements.
**Time line:** At the end of Session 5

## Preassignment

Exploration of concerns and selection using form PPS–1. Optional reading assignment is Introduction and Chapters 1 and 2 of textbook. Distribute 1 week prior to Session 1.

I. Session 1: 75 minutes, required of all staff
   A. Content and activities: emphasis is experiential learning
      1. Explore concerns as a large group and briefly discuss exploration after all concerns are generated based on preassignment.
      2. Discuss selection and shared weighting technique. Have participants perform shared weighting on 3 concerns generated during group.
      3. Introduce and discuss goals. Have participants generate 3 general goal statements for major concern identified through shared weighting.
      4. Introduce and discuss goal specification. Have participants choose 1 general goal and specify.
      5. At conclusion
         a. Collect preassignments and goal statements generated during session
         b. Announce tentative schedule for remaining sessions and voluntary participation. Registration procedures for remaining sessions.
   B. Instructional aids
      1. Easel pad
      2. Marking pens
      3. Masking tape
      4. Chalkboard
   C. Instructor activities between Sessions 1 and 2
      1. Review participants' preassignments and goal statements. Critique and return.
      2. Identify 3 clusters from participants' goal statements.
      3. Complete PPS–1G (PPS–2 or PPS–3).
      4. Prepare handout for Session 2 that indicates goal clusters, instructor's short-term goals, and tentative remaining schedule.
II. Session 2: 90 minutes
   A. Instructor's short-term goal
      1. What: participants will be able to write a specific goal relevant to expressed concerns

    2. Where/when: during class

    3. Degree: so that goal meets requirements of specification

    4. Time line: by the completion of Session 2

B. Content and activities

    1. Provide copies of all handouts or refer to tables in text (Tables 2–2 to 2–8).

       a. Participants' and instructor's goals and tentative schedule

       b. Program Planning Sheet–1

       c. Patient Participation Scale (Table 2–1)

    2. Review goal/schedule handout, which includes clusters of course goals generated from participants.

       a. Effectively involve patients with cognitive difficulties in treatment.

       b. Motivate patients.

       c. Set realistic goals.

    3. Participants individually complete Program Planning Sheet–1 relative to homework assignment 1 of interviewing patients.

    4. Group discusses Program Planning Sheet responses.

    5. Introduce and discuss Patient Participation Scale.

    6. Show videotape of interview and have participants evaluate outcomes achieved relative to their goals for impending patient interviews.

    7. At conclusion

       a. Collect individual Program Planning Sheets.

       b. Review homework assignment; distribute extra Program Planning Sheets.

C. Instructional aids

    1. Handouts

    2. Easel pad

    3. Masking tape

    4. Marker pens

    5. Videotape

    6. Videotape player and monitor

    7. Chalkboard

D. Instructor activities between Sessions 2 and 3

    1. Review collected materials.

    2. Complete PPS–2 or PPS–3.

## Homework Assignment 1

Review book section that distinguishes between goals and means; conduct at least 2 patient interviews using Program Planning Sheet–1. Read Chapter 3 of textbook.

III. Session 3: 90 minutes
    A. Instructor's short-term goal
        1. What: participants will be able to identify results/outcomes relative to their practice with patients
        2. When/where: from current clinical case load
        3. Degree: so that they can list at least 3 outcomes with the best outcome stated to meet the 4 criteria of specificity
        4. Time line: by the completion of Homework Assignment 2
    B. Content and activities
        1. Review instructor's goal from Session 2 and homework assignment. What did participants accomplish?
           a. Write a specific goal relevant to the patient's concern.
           b. State level of patient participation in defining patient goals.
        2. Introduce today's goal—outcomes and new form.
           a. List 3 outcomes for *your* use of the planning process.
           b. Select most important outcome.
           c. Specify most important outcome.
           d. Establish time line.
           e. Use documentation; handout of examples using SOAP format.
        3. Have participants address their concerns now.
        4. At conclusion
           a. Collect forms completed by participants during class.
           b. Review Homework Assignment 2 and distribute necessary forms.
    C. Instructional aids
        1. Handouts
        2. Easel pad
        3. Masking tape
        4. Marking pens
    D. Instructor activities between Sessions 3 and 4
        1. Review participants' assignments. Critique and return.
        2. Complete PPS–2 or PPS–3.

## Homework Assignment 2

1. Follow-up interviews with 3 patients; if last week's patients are available, explore outcomes of last week's goals.
2. Schedule 1 of these interviews with 1 of the instructors as an observer.
3. Use either PPS–1 or PPS–2, as appropriate, and hand in at interview with observer.
4. Bring copies of SOAP notes to next class to hand in.
5. Review Chapter 4 in textbook.

IV. Session 4: 90 minutes
   A. Goals
      1. Instructor's short-term goals with emphasis on personalization
      2. Participants' goal of involving cognitively impaired
   B. Content and activities
      1. Have participants address the following questions relative to Homework Assignment 2 (emphasize personalization).
         a. What outcomes were achieved?
         b. What worked?
         c. What concerns?
         d. What goals?
      2. Discuss application to cognitively impaired.
      3. At conclusion, review Homework Assignment 3.
   C. Instructional aids
      1. Easel pad
      2. Masking tape
      3. Marking pens
   D. Instructor: complete PPS–2 or PPS–3.

## Homework Assignment 3

Conduct daily interaction with patients as to what worked, what are the goals, what worked, and so forth, which is integral to the therapeutic setting. Write logs.

V. Session 5: 60 minutes
   A. Review of course—Patient as an independent problem solver

# References

1. DiMatteo, MR and DiNicola, DD: Achieving Patient Compliance. Pergamon Press, New York, 1982.
2. Stafford, GT: Improving patient compliance with physical therapy regimens. Unpublished paper, 1986.
3. Dishman, BK, Ickes, W, and Morgan, WP: Self-motivation and adherence to habitual physical activity. J Appl Soc Psych 10(2)115, 1980.
4. Care, GRF, Harfield, B, and Chamberlain, MA: And have you done your exercises? Physiotherapy 67(6)180, 1981.
5. Allen, VR: Follow-up study of wrist-driven flexor-hinge splint use. AM J Occup Ther 25(8)420–422, 1971.
6. Feinberg, J and Brandt, HD: Use of resting splints by patients with rheumatoid arthritis. Am J Occup Ther 35(3)173–178, 1981.
7. Seeger, MS and Fisher, LA: Adaptive equipment used in the rehabilitation of hip arthroplasty patients. Am J Occup Ther 36(8)503–508, 1982.
8. Stafford: op cit.
9. Windom, PA: The preparedness of the patient to play an active role in physical therapy in the rehabilitation setting. Unpublished master's thesis, Virginia Commonwealth University, 1979.
10. Taylor, DP: Treatment goals for quadriplegic and paraplegic patients. Am J Occup Ther 28(1)22–29, 1974.
11. Ozer, MN: The Management of Persons with Spinal Cord Injury. Demos Publications, New York, 1988, Chapter 1.
12. Matheson, LN: Work Capacity Evaluation. Employment Rehabilitation Institute of California, Anaheim, CA, 1987, p 1–11.
13. Napier, J: Hands. Pantheon Books, New York, 1980, pp 23–24.
14. Payton, OD and Ivey, JE: The role of psychoeducation in allied health practice and education. J Allied Health 10:91, 1981.
15. Martin, JE and Tubbert, PM: Behavioral management strategies for improving health and fitness. J Cardiac Rehab 4:200, 1984.
16. Rogers, JC and Figone, JJ: Psychosocial parameters in treating the person with quadriplegia. Am J Occup Ther 33(7)432–439, 1979.
17. Payton, OD: Psychosocial Aspects of Clinical Practice. Churchill-Livingstone, New York, 1986.
18. Wright, BA: Physical Disability: A Psychological Approach. Harper & Row, New York, 1960.
19. Wolf, SL (ed): Clinical Decision Making in Physical Therapy. FA Davis, Philadelphia, 1985.
20. Trombly, CA: Occupational Therapy for Physical Dysfunction, ed. 2. William & Wilkins, Baltimore, 1983.

21. Rothstein, JM and Echternach, JL: Hypothesis-oriented algorithm for clinicians: A method for evaluation and planning. Phys Ther 66:1388–1394, 1986.
22. Weed, LL: Medical Records, Medical Education and Patient Care. Case Western Reserve University Press, Cleveland, 1971.
23. Ozer, MN: A participatory planning process for wheelchair selection. In Choosing a Wheelchair System. J Rehab Res Dev Clin Suppl 2, 1989.

# Glossary

**Compliance:** obedience to orders

**Concerns / problems:** questions, needs, or complaints elicited from patients/students

**Disability:** functional or behavioral consequence of impairments

**Exploration:** the process of eliciting concerns and goals from patients/ students without critiquing responses

**Goal:** end, outcome; the result one seeks to have happen

**Impairment:** anatomic or physiologic consequence of injury or illness

**Interactive problem solving:** the process by which one involves the patient in the definition of the problem, the decisions about goals, and the evaluation of the efficacy of treatment

**Major concern:** the most important need or complaint selected from the patient/student's generated list using either prioritizing or shared weighting

**Maximum participation:** patient/student involvement at the level of free choice (level A), whenever possible. When this is not possible, movement to a lower level should occur one level at a time (multiple choice [B], forced choice [C], no choice [D]) with the patient/student's permission

**Means:** procedures, actions, measures, methods; the how of accomplishing the goal

**Outcome:** result or accomplishment

**Plan:** the combination of goal, means, and time line

**Preponderance:** the number or strength of patient concerns and goals versus those of the therapists

**Selection:** the process of identifying a major concern or goal

**Specification:** the operationalization of concern, goal, outcome, and what worked statements to include the criteria of what, when/where, and degree

**3P Method:** patient participation in planning

**Time line:** the time by which a goal is to be accomplished; the duration of time that is to elapse before the results will be accomplished and evaluation will continue

**Weighting:** a process of selecting priorities from alternatives

# Index

A page number in *italics* indicates a figure. A "t" following a page number indicates a table.

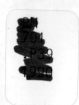